"*Yoga Radicals* is an inspiring ⟨
many leaders in modern yoga tł
these healing stories warm the heart and remind us that we are all on
journey together."

—Dr. Lori Rubenstein Fazzio, DPT, C-IAYT, Clinical Professor of Yoga and Health, Loyola Marymount University, CEO of Mosaic Physical Therapy

"Curiosity, calm, clarity, compassion, co-evolution...themes from wise souls whose practices for learning and living support our best selves and wellbeing for all. Their stories embody inspiration and possibility. As a student of systems change, I trust the body's wisdom more deeply now. Read these stories to sweeten your meditation practice."

—Peggy Holman, author of *Engaging Emergence: Turning Upheaval into Opportunity* and co-author of *The Change Handbook*

"Allie Middleton is a remarkable human. She integrates her deep study of Eastern and Western traditions in a way that is both unique and accessible. In this book, she brings together a broad spectrum of clear voices and inspired teachings. Through these brilliant, evocative interviews, she offers readers practical and poetic guidance for the realization of a better world."

—Tim Hurson, author of *Think Better*

"I have often thought of yoga as 'gentle stretching' and in fact, one practitioner near me, a physical education teacher in a public school, chose to call it that after being forbidden to use yoga in her classes. This book and the fun, inspiring stories within it, is about a different kind of gentle stretching. About a form of expanding potential. About innovation, both incremental and radical, by those using yoga to make a new or improved difference—stretching the boundaries of the possible. Whether you are a yoga teacher, individual practitioner or just a curious polymath, the diverse and inspirational stories in this book will stretch and inspire you to an expanded view of the possibilities that humans create when they have a deep care to affect the world in a positive way."

—Bob Eckert, CEO of New & Improved, LLC, New York

"*Yoga Radicals* is an inspiring, deeply informative collection of stories from a diverse group of yoga leaders. Each chapter is an individual account of transformation and a reflection on the path to wellbeing. Together, they provide light and practical guidance to a world struggling to find a better way forward. Highly recommended."

—Truett Black, Coaching and Training Director at True Development, Ltd., Taiwan

"Over the past 20 years or so, practicing yoga has become almost mainstream, but plunging deeper and committing to the vocation of yoga teacher or yoga therapist remains, indeed, an act of profound and radical love. The world is waking to a need for new paradigms—new ways of knowing that are not only actionable but also provide a springboard for the leaps of consciousness necessary to tackle the most pressing social, environmental and geopolitical issues of the day. The Yoga Radicals who've shared their stories in these pages are the mavericks who embody the paradigms that will lead our cultures forward towards futures that are not only more sustainable, but also more compassionate, and more human. This book offers stunning vistas into these futures."

—Kristine Weber, MA, c-IAYT, eRYT500, founder of Subtle Yoga, North Carolina

"For many years Allie and I have shared creativity conferences, connected at conventions and meetings designed to apply imagination and creative innovation practices to different contexts. She's one of those rare people who can take you to places you would never go. In this book she has curated stories of innovators that are invaluable. Together now in community, we might come to understand how to try something new."

—Matteo Catullo, Pathfinder, Catullo & Sylwan Advertising Agency, Creative Convergence: "How to Create the Creative Climate and Look Again," Milan

"In this eclectic collection of stories from people who practice and teach yoga from such varied perspectives, most of us will find at least one, if not more, that we resonate with. Even better is the surprise—yoga can lead to...that? Allie Middleton uncovers for us a thread whispering through the different voices: 'go ahead, try it! You have no idea where the process of the practice can take you.'"

—Jana Spalding, MD, CPSS

Yoga
Radicals

of related interest

Holding Space
The Creative Performance and Voice
Workbook for Yoga Teachers
Sarah Scharf
Foreword by Judith Hanson Lasater
ISBN 978 1 84819 405 2
eISBN 978 0 85701 361 3

**Restorative Yoga for Ethnic and
Race-Based Stress and Trauma**
Gail Parker
Forewords by Octavia F. Raheem and Amy Wheeler
Illustrated by Justine Ross
ISBN 978 1 78775 185 9
eISBN 978 1 78775 186 6

Yoga and Science in Pain Care
Treating the Person in Pain
Edited by Neil Pearson, Shelly Prosko and Marlysa Sullivan
Foreword by Timothy McCall
ISBN 978 1 84819 397 0
eISBN 978 0 85701 354 5

Yoga Therapy as a Creative Response to Pain
Matthew J. Taylor
Foreword by John Kepner
ISBN 978 1 84819 356 7
eISBN 978 0 85701 315 6

Yoga Radicals

A Curated Set of Inspiring Stories

from Pioneers in the Field

Allie Middleton

Foreword by Amy Wheeler

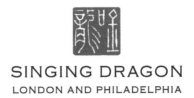

SINGING DRAGON

LONDON AND PHILADELPHIA

First published in Great Britain in 2021 by Singing Dragon,
an imprint of Jessica Kingsley Publishers
An Hachette Company

1

A CIP catalogue record for this title is available from the
British Library and the Library of Congress

ISBN 978 1 78775 467 6
eISBN 978 1 78775 468 3

Printed and bound in the United States by Integrated Books International

Jessica Kingsley Publishers' policy is to use papers that are natural,
renewable and recyclable products and made from wood grown in
sustainable forests. The logging and manufacturing processes are expected
to conform to the environmental regulations of the country of origin.

Jessica Kingsley Publishers
Carmelite House
50 Victoria Embankment
London EC4Y 0DZ

www.singingdragon.com

You are what your deep, driving desire is.
As your desire is, so is your will.
As your will is, so is your deed.
As your deed is, so is your destiny.

Brihadaranyaka Upanishad IV.4.5

We are what our deep, driving desires are.
As our desires are, so is our will.
As our will is, so are our deeds.
As our deeds are, so is our destiny.

*Now, embodying a sense of collective will:
moving from a "me" consciousness to a "we" consciousness.*

Contents

Dedication

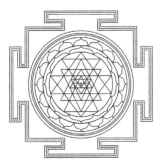

This project dedicates itself to you and to the entire field aligned with yoga, to all practitioners from time immemorial. Together, these stories celebrate the wonders and the powers, health and love that contemplative practice brings. We bow to all through time and space who benefit from ancient teachings and practices as the wisdom traditions re-root on our beloved planet now during "corona time," initiating a path for us all to experience moving from a *"me"* consciousness to a *"we"* consciousness as we renew our heartfelt cares and share in the enchantment of conscious sacred activism for the sake of the whole.

The Yoga Vidya Yantra becomes an appropriate illustration for this journey. The Shri Vidya Yantra presents a method, a philosophy, an opportunity, a path, entered into by the curious, the compassionate and the brave. Herewith an invitation to those ready for more profound inspiration from stories told by pioneers in the yoga field.

Archaeological evidence proves the appearance of rocks carved during Paleolithic times, containing images of squares holding circles, surrounding center triangles inscribed before writing, before time, as we understand and reckon with it today. Those rocks show geometric designs seemingly embedded in our human co-evolution, the collective psyche and the discovery of our own (shared) consciousness.

The Shri Vidya Yantra depicts creation, nature, and the truth in it and in us as human beings, evident after it truly reveals itself. It is profound. As you concentrate on the form and on these stories, you may see, feel and sense a taste of transformation in three sacred dimensions: Mount Meru—home of the gods and the place where the earth emerged. Keep looking at the Yantra—you can see it as a force: energy soaring upward and simultaneously descending downward. Keep watching how the points where lines intersect become a bindi, a spot, dot or point. Light shines through them at each intersection of the bindi. Two bindis connect each other in a line, three make a surface, a fourth adds the wonder of space. It fills out into a complex yet orderly design which holds and continuously reveals the truth emerging about the elements, the chakras, our emerging knowledge of our star-filled Cosmos and similarly stardust-filled Self.

And as you now settle and sense into the path behind the stories shared here, we trust that a recognition of the potential of further seeding and way-finding will inspire your aspiration, perhaps to listen more deeply to the guidance contained here and within the All and Everything.

Amy Kline Gage

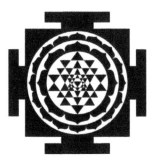

Refuge Weavers

Guardians of the light
with hearts as healer
spines as support
now rooted in earth
together;
breath as intimate touchstone
welcoming energies within
and without,
together.

The new score emerges
aligning and attuning to
what is around
up and down
inside and out
and all around.
We are all together.
We sit to stand
to lie down
to travel
through time and space,
together.

New rhythms unraveling the old,
unweaving patterns and
welcoming new treasures,
together.

Foreword

Yoga Radicals grows from a seed planted by Allie Middleton when she envisioned the co-creative process of curating the narratives for this book. Allie conceived of the idea when she was a presenter for a panel session at the International Association of Yoga Therapists annual conference. The topic was Social Activism and Community Healing.

Allie applied the Theory U prototyping models for her interview process and crafted a "Presencing Approach" with each author. She helped the authors pull ideas out of the ether, and to bring them into a form where we can all enjoy and delight in them. These chapters outline how each author embodies a positive "life force" and uses it to do good in the world, according to their personal values, beliefs and perceptions. The authors exemplify how to follow the path of yoga. That is to say that each author is connected to something deep inside, and they move in a direction that is in alignment with the still and subtle voice that is whispering to them. It is from each author's link to Self, that the creative force has emerged as a unique life's work offering.

This book was formed during the "global pause" that we experienced as a yoga community during the lockdown from COVID-19 in 2020. During the lockdown many of us saw our life habits and patterns, as well as our inner energies, shifted and re-organized. We collectively saw that the field of yoga also had a chance to pull back, get quiet, re-think and redesign who we are as a yoga family and how we desire to impact the world we live in. This great pause gave us a chance to examine our duties, our relationship to the divine, to human laws, to community, to family, and to Self. I would argue that COVID-19 gifted us a precious and rare opportunity to come together and co-create a new trajectory for our future.

Before the pandemic, the yoga industrial complex was not really working for the common yoga teacher who was running too fast and not able to make ends meet energetically or financially. It appeared that many yoga teachers and yoga therapists had fallen into the trap of trading true internal power for faux external power in hopes for a chance at survival. Many of us had bought into capitalism, consumerism, hierarchy, patriarchy, cultural appropriation, unconscious and conscious racism. We were also carrying the heavy burden of the shame that accompanies the surrender of our yamas and niyamas. The pandemic pause, "corona time," has helped us to ask the hard questions we often dismiss: "What did I ignore?", "Where am I complicit?", "Where are my blind spots?", "Where am I not being courageous?", and finally "What does my mind and body need to stay in balance so that I can live an honest life, offering practices for equitable wellbeing and from a place of clarity?"

The first step of gaining clarity is to have an attitude of detachment toward our attachments, aversions, ego identifications, misperceptions and fears. Then we are able to move in a new direction toward the light of higher consciousness. It follows that as we each tend to our own inner light we will inspire each other, and we will play off the impact of one another's ideas and actions. The "I" will become the "We." It is even possible that because of the deconstruction and reconstruction of the yoga world during 2020, we might finally realize that there never was an "I." It has always been the "We." It is my hope that this book will facilitate moving our minds and hearts in the direction of the We.

Amy Wheeler, Ph.D.
April 2021

Acknowledgments

I am deeply indebted to all the teachers and wisdom traditions from all of Nature who stand here on the planet with us now as we co-evolve.

Many at the International Association of Yoga Therapists have been instrumental in this work, supportive and encouraging. Thank you all.

Deep gratitude to the Singing Dragon team at Jessica Kingsley Publishers for seeing the potential of unearthing these stories.

With deep thanks to readers in my family and friendship network who listened and danced with me as I journeyed through this process. Special thanks to James Dixon in Glasgow for essential support, and to my beloved Newell for sharing the journey and nourishing the joy of our love.

To "corona time" for helping us all wake up.

I bow to the many Yoga Radicals whose embodied stories will yet be told as they unfold.

And to the abundant and magnificent All and Everything who helps keep us wondering.

Preface

These narratives contain the actual words from hour-long dialogues, with a few grammatical edits. Of course, they are much shorter, but I hope they capture the essence of each Yoga Radical. They emerge from an open-hearted sense of inquiry and are grounded in shared sacred practice, a sense of deep shared essence, a quality we might call resting-in-being. They provide a structured reminder of the truth and beauty and goodness of the forces that emerge from consistent reflection, inquiry and practice, regardless of history or context. My hope in grounding the questions and the narratives in a transformative dialogue engagement practice is to help to reveal a conscious activation and renewal process of embodied presence practices. Together, may they serve to offer a broad and general set of revelations that weave together a curious, compassionate and courageous potential of a more embodied future.

Should you wish to access a few samples of the full interview transcripts, they can be downloaded from https://library.singingdragon.com/redeem using the code WHCRVZE.

Our emerging future depends on yoga therapy and other mind–body integration practices to become integral aspects of our communities, organizations, families and teams so we might have a chance to protect and sustain the wellbeing of us all during this time of great change.

The personal stories are evidence that we are emerging from the shock of "corona time" transformed. Each is moving yet connected to something eternal; listen for that. Each Yoga Radical story demonstrates the impact of devoted personal practice. These diverse leaders have each found ways to expand the benefits cultivated from the soil of their own personal practice and to transplant it to seed in the collective soil for our greater good.

This is what we are seeking: an embodied collective aspirational view into our future potential, here crystallized in a set of curated presencing-inspired narratives, true models from the ancient art of alchemy. I hope you too will feel how this golden collective blend forms seeds for a transformational new rootedness in contemplative inquiry. These Yoga Radicals (and the many others out there on the planet...) are stars of grounded practice. They each contain the imprint of embodied potentiality now being seeded and further cultivated during this epochal collective shift on the planet as we move from "*me*" to "*we*" consciousness.

I approach this with deep appreciation of all my teachers, guides and angels along the way.

Let us thank them all with a deep bow, and may their actions inspire us all to act from our shared cosmic heart for the sake of our species and our beloved planet.

We are all wayfinders now; keep listening and welcoming the ancient goodness and wisdom from all directions.

Love in the Dark Matter

(...songs to silence...as we move from *"me"* to *"we"*...)

Mending and tending the tears in the tapestry
our existence breaks apart;
we are connecting to the earth body again.
All colors and energies uniting in solid bands,
ribbons streaming and steaming us
forward now
as we sit and meditate.
Alone, yet together,
oh joy!
All our bodies and their riotous confluences
now flowing and flowering though all through the waterways
even while weighted with the ever-burning embers of
transformation.
Might we finally greet each other as "One";
spacious elements all around and in us as one?
Air bound and earthbound and fire and space bound,
floating again in shared existence, our waters now clear
and breathing usefully and
at once, simultaneously,
we sing,
hallelujah!
as the new ones emerge in peaceful union.

Introduction

The concept for this work evolved from the inaugural Common Interest Community forum on Community Healing and Social Activism at SYTAR 2018, a conference hosted by the International Association of Yoga Therapists (IAYT). I was invited by Matthew Taylor to work with Lilith Bailey-Kroll to combine some of our interests and co-facilitate the inaugural Common Interest Community on Community Healing and Social Activism.

Many emerging yoga leaders responded to our request for proposals. Six were chosen to participate. I was excited to work collaboratively through the process with other yoga therapists at the International Association of Yoga Therapists to mount a half-day event to hear the stories of how dedicated yoga practice opened a pathway to innovations that initiated community healing and social activism.

To structure the inquiry of moving from a *"me"* focus to a *"we"* focus, we employed Joseph Campbell's Hero/Heroine's Journey model as a basis to bring the dharma stories to life. I blended that personal approach with a more systems-based approach from the Presencing Institute (www.presencing.org). The star-shaped prototyping model formed the perfect mudra for our investigation into embodied change-making. Our collective journey evolved; we were all on fire about how to co-initiate a new embodied conversation, a conscious dialogue that unearths the genius of yoga-inspired innovation from leaders in the emerging yoga therapy space.

After the conference, the project grew into a year-long refinement comprised of group video conference calls to deepen and broaden the awareness-based change process. Narratives were curated and subsequently published in IAYT-sponsored blogs and feature magazine articles as the project grew and took on its own momentum.

For this current project, I was invited to source yoga-based innovation further, to interview dozens of global yoga leaders from all places and spaces, each with a staggering wealth and diversity of experience and leadership capacity to begin to further flesh out this emerging landscape of collective intelligence: personal articulations of embodied awareness in social activism and community healing. These Yoga Radicals are the spontaneous creators of innovation as well as more senior representatives of multigenerational practice environments. They are the current flock of free agents who have metabolized this unique offer to the emerging profession of yoga therapy. Each agreed to sing their embodied song: theirs is the job of bringing the process of transformative yoga-based practices forward into the collective. Their gifts bring simple and complex living human treasures to our co-evolving world and will serve the wellbeing of humanity and the emerging profession of yoga therapy.

My heart's desire is to share these jewels of yoga-based leadership and wisdom in the hope that these stories will nourish your practice as well as further cultivate your interest in contributing to the growing field of yoga therapy for the sake of our planet, now more than ever in need of embodied presence and transformative leadership.

As you read the stories, the thoughts and experiences contained in these pages, you may find yourself surprised, as each and every one is illuminating in very different ways. Trust the intention of these Yoga Radicals as they sing their songs of passion and practice, such abundant material for you to take with you as you walk your own path, wherever you find yourself on your journey.

Through these interviews and conversations, you will find something that is simultaneously very specific and very nebulous, obvious yet hard to pin down, entirely universal yet deeply personal. You may also discover how a deep commitment to personal practice can inspire something new to be born on a larger scale.

As I was getting ready for this project, I was finishing a book of a first collection of poems, some of which are sprinkled through this work. They are poems that emerged over the decades after meditation or while on retreat in nature. Similarly, the interview process was designed to be a shared aesthetic experience of shared embodied presence practice. Each moment embraced a space of deep focused attention and intention to be present in sacred time with the numinous, the non-dual, the ever-emerging eternal. Each is anchored in a deep bliss of connection to ancient teachings and their perennial wisdom as well as illuminated with fresh seeing, feeling and sensing.

The interviews were conducted virtually between April and August 2020, as everyone on the planet was adapting to "corona time." These stories have become available now because of our shared dedication to deepening our practices, telling our stories from the intelligence of the heart. May these seeds of transformation invite flourishing and invoke inspiration for the emergence of a new collective will for healing and wellbeing for all. Let us continue to cultivate and nourish the golden threads of ancient wisdom transmitted here.

These yogis, these thinkers, these feelers, each a "moving-from-me-to-we seeker," have gifted us insights and linkages to a deepening capacity for ongoing personal transformation while activating and participating in the emergence of a new collective unfolding. As awareness practices open the space for something new, we see, we feel and we sense how we might all restore and renew ancient wisdom practices to inspire fresh ways of living, learning, working and loving together. The wisdom flowing through these stories shows us, in part, how efficiently and effectively we might all learn to listen deeply and to welcome change. Our senses are seeking something entirely fresh and novel, making time and space for extraordinary wellbeing and harmony. In this collective dance of honoring, we re-member the fragments of the ancient truths, embodying and reintegrating the roots of our shared human becoming; we are breathing life in and releasing what no longer serves our promising potential of divine collective unfolding.

Reader's guide
The curation process: how it worked

My task was simple enough in its own way, if daunting. These yoga innovators live all around the world, so I scheduled video conference calls for all of our interviews. Then came the laborious process of transcription, of parsing each interview to secure the golden nuggets of wisdom, lived experience and transmission they each contain. This was breathtaking, navigating the wisdom and insight so as to let the embodied presence of the words shape into a representative body of prose to fit into an experience of an interview practice and conscious dialogue process. As you have also embarked on this journey, feel free to skip around. Wherever you find yourself on your path, we must trust that somewhere here you will find nuggets to treasure and savor, to help you move forward on your contemplative journey.

Authorship in this way is a pleasure and an aesthetic curatorial labor, like writing poetry or mounting a gallery exhibition in a museum or library. However, as many of the Yoga Radicals here have made clear, most forms of practice that enable an activation of embodied presence offer full, creative views of a type of wholesome clarity, sometimes even with a light-hearted awareness. I hope you might also dare to take a similar step (or skip!) on your path of contemplative inquiry and embodied action. Now, this collective journey we are all experiencing on the planet during "corona time" requires patience and perseverance. There really is no escaping the reality of how important attention and intention practices are, as we navigate in this changed world. Yet, at this stage, I also wanted to have some fun and share being-ness with these amazing yoga innovators, each so generously sharing the energy of an emerging collective awareness in the early spring of 2020. That is what I hope for you, too. As the saying goes, "We are all in this together!"

The inquiry itself is fairly simple, I suppose. The basis of everything I am seeking can be summed up as follows:

How might the impact of sustained personal contemplative practices initiate a deeper focus with expanded awareness that activates a new global capacity to co-evolve, seeding the discovery of emerging multi-level innovations that serve wellbeing and harmony for all?

Every aspect of the inquiry includes a combination of a personal healing journey on the way to transforming into a flourishing social innovation for the sake of something greater. Each and every question, every minor conversation branched off from this central pursuit. It was a sustained corona-inspired reflective blend of curiosity, compassion and courage. I was seeking to find the sensitivity and serenity to release judgment and cynicism and fear so that the light and truth of each Yoga Radical might shine forth.

Inspiration is just the seed of potential. What is offered here is a sense of shared being-ness, a collection of embodied true natures that may have sufficient impact to initiate real change on the ground, for the earth, for our bodies and the emerging social body, using the intelligence of the mind and heart as well as conscious embodiment of ancient practices that we love so well. The soil of our yoga-inspired field is rich and new seeds need cultivation now. It's as if the practices are loving us back as we learn to listen, re-member and restore the primary importance of reflective inquiry on the planet today. Realizing this is a contemplative leadership journey in itself, we are re-engaging and re-enchanting the ancient forms of conscious attention and awareness practices to help ideas land and locate into a conscious collective landing strip for our co-evolution into a positive shared future. Listening deeply now and inviting, now invoking, the personal body, the earth body and conscious social bodies to breathe us back into a harmonious whole being. Restoring our faith in humanity, one Yoga Radical story at a time, let these stories inspire us. So now, you might ask yourself, what might my ideal future be and how might I take the stories to heart as I continue breathing right here now, on the path, in this journey of this body's life on earth? You can start cultivating your own meaningful project with others, no matter how large or small. Most of all, enjoy the journey as it unfolds. Let the magic delight you and hold you close.

Ultimate Expansion

emanating from the center
we hope for peace
we release fear
stepping toward freedom

light guides us
creating more rays of light
we discover the space
of new beginnings.

enjoy how the mystery and stillness opens
communities of passion and love

new perspectives arising
we recognize
the space of listening
more deeply
to each other

and ourselves.

here a pathway
of innocence arises

a new vision is
looking again
toward new life

a creation place
for
deep caring

ultimate expansion,
ultimate potential.

Homage to Pythagoras

If our particulars create a shape
as we listen to the music of the spheres

what magic streams through?

Is it me, is it thee, is it we, or is it something quite else...

Where did we ever get this notion of existence?

As such, and nonetheless, it seems

we must enter the dance of forever...

together.

Yoga
Radicals

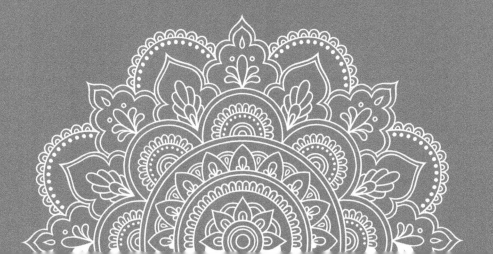

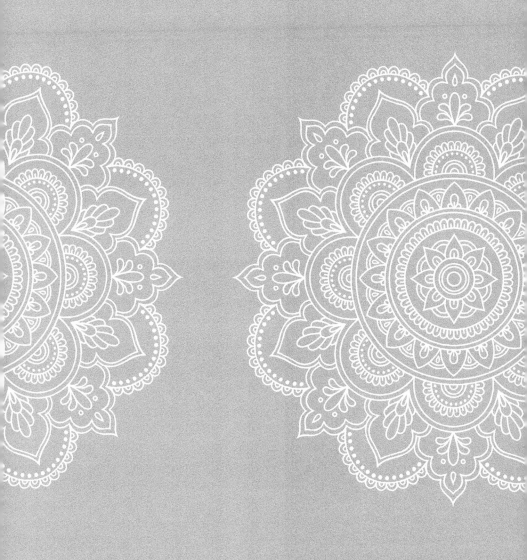

I

The Journey Starts

Arriving with Deeper Listening

*Stories about transforming
perception, gathering attention,
mindfulness, extending awareness.*

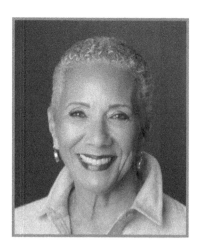

• • • • •

Gail Parker is a psychologist, author and educator. She is the author of *Restorative Yoga for Ethnic and Race-Based Stress and Trauma*, a first-of-its-kind book that describes how Restorative Yoga can be used as an effective self-care tool that helps you navigate the stresses and traumas arising from daily lived experiences associated with race.

She is well known for her pioneering efforts to blend psychology, yoga and meditation as effective self-care strategies that can enhance emotional balance and contribute to the overall health and wellbeing of practitioners. Her broad expertise in behavioral health and wellness includes 40 years as a practicing psychotherapist and 20 years as a yoga therapy educator. She has been a featured psychology expert on nationally and internationally syndicated talk shows including numerous appearances on *The Oprah Show*. She is the President of the Black Yoga Teachers Alliance Board of Directors.

Gail Parker

If people need a formula, now's the time to think about who you've been. To think about who you are in this moment of crisis and trauma and stress. All of us don't know ourselves in trauma and stress. And we're all in trauma and stress right now. We just are. So who am I now, and who do I want to become? That's our future, now's the time.

I've been practicing yoga for 50 years. A class was being offered at my local art institute. And I think I went out of curiosity; that was the driver. Curiosity brought me. I didn't have a commitment to yoga or anything like it.

It was probably more like what we would call Yoga Nidra now, where we would go do a body scan and just relax. That was the practice. I remember feeling it was during a time of great turmoil and upheaval for a lot people in the United States of America, the peak of the civil rights movement in the midst of the riots that took place in urban centers.

I remember this experience as a peace and calm that came over me. That was profound. And as I'm talking about this, I'm remembering my grandmother who was the presence of peace and calm always; nothing seemed to shake her up. I remember as a little girl, I would just look at her and wonder about that and wonder how that was and wish and want that for myself.

The class was held once a week, and on Sundays the teacher gave lectures about self-realization. He gave us a book that was written by Paramahansa Yogananda, *Autobiography of a Yogi*, which went way over my head, but I tried to read it.

That was how I started. I didn't have a clue about who was teaching the yoga, about who Mr. Black really was. It was not until, I would say, within the past ten years that I found out who he was. I stumbled upon this knowledge. I realized, "Oh, I was introduced to yoga by a master," which is why I kept the practice up. I think I only took his classes for a year because for some reason they were disbanded, and then there was no other place to go.

So you'd get a book, you'd look at the picture, you do the pose and that was your yoga.

I learned from the beginning an advanced form of practice, which is a home practice, doing it on one's own, which of necessity involved discipline, self-study and this connection with a higher power.

That would be Kriya Yoga. And that's in fact what he was teaching. Mr. Black was a direct disciple of Paramahansa Yogananda. I did not know that at the time, I found that out, as I said; it was just miraculous the way that unfolded. I was inspired by the practice and maybe I was inspired to go to that art institute in the first place. That was the experience of it.

I suspect the seed was planted long before yoga. As a child, I was always deeply inspired. I had a deep connection to spiritual practices. That was always in me and always moving me.

"You seem so wise; where does that come from?" I don't know. There has been a connection to that wisdom body, which again is part of our yoga practice as well. When you start studying it, you learn that there is such a thing, and so I've always been in, if not consciously aware of that, some way that's always moved through me.

I don't know how I have always known that I had an inner life. I always knew it from the time I was a little, little girl and I always called on it. I always called on it and it never failed me. I know how to do that. I don't know how I know how to do that. I don't know how I know how to say, "Take a moment, take a breath, check within."

I remember one time I was miserable; I was absolutely desolate, and I was in fear in my life. I remember standing in the front of my window, overlooking the river where I lived at the time, just forlorn. I didn't know what to do. I didn't know where to turn. And all of a sudden there's voice saying to me, "So what would you tell your clients to do?"

I said to myself, "No wonder they get so mad at me, because I didn't want to do what I myself said to do." I did. And I thought, "Oh, no wonder they don't like it when I tell them that stuff." So I did it.

Awareness. See, you can have that gift without awareness. Awareness comes with wisdom, real wisdom, not the wisdom... Little kids can say things that sound very wise, but there's not awareness. I remember my son saying to me once when he was four, "You know what, Mommy? Life doesn't die." I never forgot it.

So I think you have to marry the gift with awareness, and then you can become intentional in how you apply it.

I mean, these are all circumstances I'm thinking about that I have found myself in where you go within, you get an answer. It's a real answer from that knowing space, it's what you know because your body is telling you and then you have to be intentional with what you do with it. So there's choice involved also. We have a choice.

My life took me there. I stopped planning 30 years ago. I don't make plans. I don't have agendas. When I'm in a yoga class, for example, and the instructor says, "Okay, think of your intention," I always go blank.

But by the time the practice is over, something will have come to me. All right. So again, my plan to the extent that there is one and when I can honor it, I don't always. Assuming that no one's running a perfect game here. I intentionally try to cooperate with life.

I was supposed to go back to Michigan at the end of April, in March when everything began to shut down here. I don't know how long I'll be here; if I have to stay here for the rest of the year, I will. I'm not going anywhere until life tells me to—it's that. Whatever that is, awareness is paying attention to what's going on around you, and what's going on within you and then making a choice.

Well, I have to tell, this may not be very helpful, but for me at this stage of the game, it's all over. It is not in any location in my body.

I was afraid because it was on the eve of my seventieth birthday. And I was scared because I was associating that age with death, mortality. So I had been in deep contemplation about my own mortality, my death, all of that. And I was talking to my son, we were talking, I was talking to him. And I'm waxing eloquent about mortality and this and that, and the other thing.

He looked at me, he said, "Mom, are you okay?" I said, "I'm fine." He said, "How do you feel?" I said, "I feel great." He looked at me, he said, "Exactly."

That's how I do it. I remind myself every day, especially now; every single day in the immediacy of the day I wake up and I check it out. I say, "I'm okay, I'm fine. I'm fine." I feel okay, I can breathe. I'm fine, that's how I do it.

What I do know in my heart, and hope will be true, is that when we connect with that aspect of self, that is okay, and then yoga, that would be the Anandamaya Kosha, our bliss body, which is more than a feeling of bliss. It is a sense of wellbeing, an awareness that I am more than this body. I know that I'm more than my body. I didn't always know that. I know that I'm even more than my breath—which is pretty amazing, especially during these times—more than my feelings, more than my thoughts. I am more than all of that.

It's that Westerners don't always have that awareness that my soul is primal, the primacy of soul. And one of the things that I think is lacking in the way yoga is presented in Western culture, to the extent that it is lacking, is this elimination of talk about any spirituality of soul. There's a shyness about having that conversation. Well, we don't want to offend anybody, we don't want to upset people who don't believe that, but when you begin to realize, "Wait a minute, that's who I am. I am a spiritual being, having a human experience." And you know that, and you get that, and you practice that, and you try to live into that. It's a hard concept. So conceptually, it's really hard to manage, but when you really understand that, "No, my spirit is who, that's fine."

So what does that mean? Well, we know when to send the spirit of laughter, don't we? We would call it energy. But it's the spirit of laughter. We know the spirit of sadness. We know the spirit of love. We know all of this; we use scientific language to talk about spiritual things. Like we play it safe in that respect. So for those readers who are more comfortable with scientific language, call it energy. Use the language that resonates with you, but this is what I'm calling our spirituality, our soulfulness.

When you learn in your yoga teacher training, they start with the physical body. The physical body is the hardest part or aspect of ourselves to change. It is within that other space that we have lots of room to become. That's the field of pure potentiality that you're talking about. What is that? What are you talking about? It's that willingness to live into that spiritual aspect of self—you contemplate it, you sit with it, you wonder about it. You get curious, you study it. It's all of it.

It is clear to me that I don't know what's going to happen. I don't know what the future holds. But how do you live in the not-knowing? It takes practice; if you are not clear, if you are not used to going within and listening to and cultivating a relationship with your inner voice, then you don't know.

If you hear it, if you practice listening, "Okay. Let's say I have an inner voice. Let me see what that is. Let me listen to it," and then you take a chance on listening to what it tells you to do. Remember when I said, my voice said, I don't want to do that, but I took a risk and did it anyway. It's that, you have to be willing to take the risk to act on what that inner voice is telling you. And then you make a mistake... I love that part of wisdom. A teacher of mine taught me, "If you make a mistake, don't do it again. If you do it again, don't do it again." It's that. You learn to trust your inner voice. What our yoga practices teach us is to pause and then consider our action so that we're acting from a place of clarity.

If you haven't practiced that, it's like trying to teach a drowning person how to swim. It's not a good idea. That's not a good time to teach someone how to swim. So if you were in the midst of turmoil now and you've never practiced just being still, this will be a challenge for you.

But this is a good time to do it since everybody is being invited to do it anyway, all of this acting out that we see—in yoga speak, you could call it the gunas, you can call this Rajasic energy or Tamasic energy where you're paralyzed. The Satvic energy, the sweetness of balance comes from those two out of line. We're not trying to get rid of either one. We're trying to bring that into balance.

In psychology talk, it would be "don't just do something, sit there." Wait until your nervous system comes to a place of calm, because then you can see with more clarity, and you will make better decisions from a place of clarity. That's the yoga.

That's the second sutra. We quiet the busyness of the mind first.

So this is not something that happens instantly. This takes time, energy, effort, dedication, intention, commitment and practice. And sometimes it's uncomfortable. It is hard to be still when you want to jump out of your skin, but that's the word.

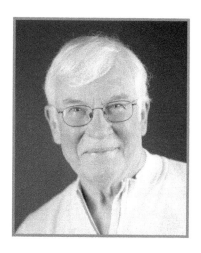

• • ● • •

Michael Lee has had a long career in yoga and yoga therapy with a focus on psycho-emotional health spanning more than three decades. Prior to coming to the USA in 1984 to pursue yoga therapy training, Michael was an academic and consultant in the behavioral sciences in Australia. He co-founded Phoenix Rising Yoga Therapy in 1986 based on his learning and integration of yoga and elements of contemporary psychology, now supported by neuroscience.

Michael is the author of *A Bridge from Body to Soul* and *Turn Stress into Bliss*. He is also a contributing author to *Beyond Talk Therapy: Using Movement and Expressive Techniques in Clinical Practice*, published by the American Psychological Association. Michael is a frequent speaker at global yoga therapy conferences. Michael and his wife, Lori, parent five adult children and live in rural Massachusetts.

Michael Lee

I've been able to engage with discernment and in many ways trust it to choose wisely, even though I haven't always chosen wisely. But it seems to me that this conditioning is what I need always to hold in my awareness during one-on-one work, in my teaching, in my training programs: to create that space where people are safe but, at the same time, challenged to embrace ways of being or trying on ways of being that potentially open to a greater awareness, a greater insight, a greater wisdom.

Probably the earliest spark that I can feel a relationship with was this deep longing for a change. The change was in a way of being that was just somehow more compatible with everything. My work actually evolved into that.

There was a lot of support for it then. Because I was living in Australia, we inherited a form of organizing ourselves in the workplace on basically a British model, which was very hierarchical. In many ways it was uncaring for human beings as unique creatures. It's basically putting round pegs into square holes and vice versa.

I could sense that. I thought, "There's got to be a better way to do this." I'd done a lot of work with places like Tavistock and Esalen, where I got the latest ideas on human behavior and change. I started to lead some programs on that. That worked pretty well, except that it was all in the head. So people would get these great ideas, wonderful ideas, "Yay, let's do this. Let's do that," but they'd go back, and, within weeks sometimes, it would die on the vine, no change really, because there was no felt sense of it. I liken it now to a switch. There's something that has to click, like a switch going off that confirms and validates, "Yes, this is how I want to be."

That went on for a while, and then one morning I stumbled into yoga. I got to a point where I got tired of going to the gym. I got tired of just going for a run. I thought, "There's got to be more." I moved into an intentional community, because we wanted to live a more in-touch-with-the-world-and-nature kind of lifestyle. It just seemed right that I should take a look at yoga. I'd learned a lot about a lot of things in the counterculture that kind of pointed in that direction—going off to meditate and stuff like that.

I ended up in an Iyengar class and thought, "Oh my god, what have I hit?"

I started a practice at home. I started to do my own practice. One morning I was practicing with my daughter. She was about nine. She was watching me practice, and, at the end, she said, "Dad, I like when you do that." I said, "Why?" She said, "When you do that stuff, you're not so grumpy." It was like a rock hit me. I could feel a different state of being when I did my practice.

I stumbled across Kripalu, which had, at that time, just moved from Pennsylvania to Massachusetts. They had a master's program. I was the only person that ever took that program. It's almost like it was created for me and no one's ever done it since.

I was totally in love with the whole thing. It was everything. It was the feel of it, the practices, the people. It was just like, "Whoa, this is a whole thing that's here to support the kind of thing that I want to do in my life. Here it is. I'm so lucky. I'm so blessed to be here." I was totally into it, even with the difficulties, like my eldest daughter not liking the food, all kinds of little things that I had to deal with, but we worked it through. We did it.

It took a while to decide, but it was just, "I'm going to stay. I'm not going back." I let go of so much, and that was the other part, too. To do this, I had to let go of a lot. I let go of tenure as a professor at a college. I let go of a salary that had fantastic vacation times, all the stuff that people would dream about. I just went back. I actually took a journey back (to Australia) and resigned.

There was one experience I had. Don Stapleton was one of my mentors. He and I were doing assisted postures with each other, and I think our intention was exploring the upper limbs of yoga and seeing how asana could connect into the upper four limbs, particularly through the four virtues or four immeasurables, the bramaviharas. I was against the wall in a triangle pose, and I got to that edge where, if I had been practicing by myself, I probably would have said, "Okay, next posture." I stayed there. There was something. That was another confirming moment. It was a leap in faith. It was kind of like a journey to an unknown place I'd never been before in my body. But with the safety that was there, the presence, the love that I could feel and that he didn't have any agenda. He wasn't trying to make me get anywhere or do anything to me. He was just being there, which he had a real good knack of being able to do, which was fantastic.

After a while, it settled down, and I felt almost blissful, like I could stay there.

That particular incident led to a very significant change in my life. After that experience, I could feel and sense my own power and my own agency to place myself any way I chose in the world, and that was scary, because, given that it was a choice, oh my god, that's an obligation now. What am I going to choose?

I think, in that moment, it was a choice for love. It was the first time in my life I'd seen that clearly. I could choose fear; I could choose love. So it was a big opening that took me further into the deeper practices. Knowing that that possibility existed at that particular moment that could possibly be embraced by just about anyone if the conditions were right.

Basically, there was a quest to set up these conditions and to learn that through my own experiences. And then finding out that my experiences didn't match other people's experiences, so I had to allow for that too, and start to see people wherever they were as being someone who, if they chose and if the conditions were right, could change, could grow, could learn, could grow in more love, have more compassion, be more open.

So I had to learn then, over the next probably 30 years, what it really was all about, and it's been a great journey, because it's just been continual letting go and opening, letting go, opening. It wasn't any accident that I called the work Phoenix Rising, because that's been my life: dying to the old and born to the new every so often. That's the journey.

The things that I started to bring into setting up the conditions in the development of my work were, in a way, outside the yoga world, and some of it was more Buddhist than yoga. It was a very non-dual process. I was aware of this not quite fitting anywhere really. We didn't fit the psychotherapy world. We didn't fit the yoga world. We weren't Buddhist monks.

Who are we? Well, who am I? But there were people being drawn to it the more I engaged myself. And I wasn't even going to teach. I was working one-on-one basically when I started this. I thought, "This is a one-on-one thing," because that's how it occurred to me in triangle posture. A lot of the development I did was around working with people one-on-one. I had some success with people where I could set up conditions that could support them going through a door of some kind and having a different experience with themselves that potentially was like transformative, not to feel the power of it, but even so it was still an oddity.

I didn't even know what to call it.

It took a while. It really did. There were many years of being on the defensive and not even knowing it, trying to fit, getting disappointed. And then I guess there was also then some real ego gratification, because once I started to teach and go broader than just the one-on-one, I was a pretty capable teacher, so it wasn't difficult for me to gather some kind of a following, but that was fraught with its ego stuff, too. I had to have a couple of experiences of crashing and burning to realize that that was the case. This wasn't about that. So when I'd engage those kinds of experiences, I'd draw back, and I'd draw back into what I knew, which really was my practice. For example, not long after I started, I went through a divorce from my first wife. I'd wake up on the mat every morning. I'd get on the mat after I woke up and I'd be in tears. And I'd just trust the practice, trust the practice.

I think what bridged me into a greater social awareness and a greater embracing of all kind of ways of being was learning about compassion. It was lacking in my life. Although I had all the other things, I could do the work, it was being sought after, it was the ego thing, it was all I had, but time and time again I'd come up against this lack of compassion, in relationships, in the way I worked, even the way I ran my organization. There was something that didn't ring true. The ideas were there. The thoughts were there. The dialogue was there. But the actual felt sense of it was missing.

It was about that time, and we're going back somewhere around ten years ago probably, where I started to develop a growing interest in Buddhism as well as yoga. I started to come across different teachings that really spoke to me. I was going through some relationship issues and I was getting some therapy, and my therapist happened to be an ex-Catholic priest who was now a Buddhist and follower of Thich Nhat Hanh, and he gave me this thing to read, I think it was a poem, in relation to my wife, Lori.

It was simply a statement of "I am here. I can't fix it. I can't change it. But I want you to know I'm here." I can't remember the exact words or the book. I think it was in *Radical Love* or something like that. It landed in my body, that whole thing of being here, which really is a lot of what my work's about, but it hadn't landed in that deeper way. And then I began to practice more in the Theravadan tradition. I sought out people that I saw as leaders in that arena who had an approach that I could really resonate with.

Just over time I started to change myself in my relationships. I think that was what it was, where I could really embrace, from a real felt sense, not just a head space. Way back when I joined an intentional community, I was doing it for the same reason, but it was up here, in my head. Gradually, as I'd kind of gone through my own work, it got deeper and deeper within me.

A sense of ease, a sense of ease with a big mystery, I guess. I dabbled a little bit in quantum theory. I don't know how to explain all that, but I can feel it. I can know that there's some truth there. It's just this is how I need to be now.

And, again, from my own experience, it's almost like I've been able to grow because there's been the freedom to grow.

One of the conditions that gives rise to insight and wisdom in a way of practicing, in a way of delivering one-on-one work, in a way of engaging, is trusting that a spark of wisdom and insight will flow outwards. It's going to affect others. No one walks away from one of our training programs, I would hope, the same being that walked in, and that difference is going to make a difference. There will be more room in their world for embracing all of it.

II

Grounding and Co-Initiating

Planting Seeds of Potential

Welcoming the emerging future
with embodied creativity.

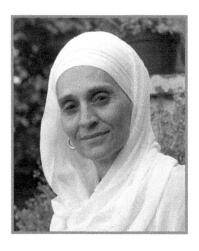

• • • • •

Itta Roussos, "Ravi," is a lead trainer and mentor registered with KRI and Yoga Alliance, and a yoga activist who trains yoga teacher trainers and yoga teachers.

Ravi founded Kundalini Africa Rising in 2015 to address social justice issues with regard to the training of yoga teachers of color in Southern Africa and elsewhere in the world. Ravi teaches and consults in addiction rehabilitation centers and counseling centers for gender-based violence and for individuals living with HIV/AIDS, and maintains a private practice. Ravi trains yoga therapists through Sat Sangat Yoga Therapy school. Ravi specializes in using yoga therapy and psychology for the healing of individual intergenerational trauma, community trauma, attachment dysfunctions, post-traumatic stress disorder and pregnancy.

Itta Roussos

So it's not an individual working within a community. It's a community of yogis. We have a mantra or a mission statement that we developed together. And it started off being the radical integration of social justice and spiritual practice. And we now have shortened it, and we say social justice is a spiritual practice. And that is really what we use to inform everything that we do. As a community, we come together using the practice for the purpose of social justice. Not only, although that's a byproduct for personal enlightenment, but just for the enlightenment of all.

I grew up in a very small, very conservative town in the days of apartheid. In those days, the church dominated the people, which was very separate from the white people who lived in the village. Black people lived completely separately, outside of the village, and served as the labor pool. My first exposure to yoga was a woman called Jewel whom I knew for six months. She then disappeared and I've never ever seen her again. I was 12. She was so inspiring to me that her interests lasted the rest of my life. She left after six months because the church threatened to excommunicate the people who were attending her classes, all women. So they all stopped going to her classes. So Jewel left because she couldn't make a living. Her teaching lived on in me. Now it lives on in the many people whose lives I've touched. So that was my first inspiration. I started working as a yoga teacher at the age of 20, because I'd been practicing on my own. And right from that time, in South Africa, along with the rest of Africa, the "*we*" is a very present concept if we allow it to be here.

So it was always the "*we*" that inspired my path.

And all of the philosophy that I studied on my own at the time, it was also about service. So I started teaching as an activist. I started teaching activists who were getting burned out, suffering from PTSD, really because of being arrested and tortured and in hiding and on the run. I was so enamored with how healthy and alive and vital yoga kept me that I made a commitment to teach activists how to do self-care. This was in the late seventies and early eighties in the middle of the worst times of apartheid.

I feel that I can't be happy if you're not happy. That's the principle of Ubuntu.

And that is what is so powerful here on the African continent. Still on this continent, even though there is still so much colonization and so much abuse of Africa, not all the people here feel it. It's still such a powerful and aligned community aspect. And community includes the earth.

And the people that I was working with were not white. Yoga was always seen as a practice that belongs only to white people. So it took me a long time to gather enough energy in my personal practice and to have people trust me. That it isn't a religion, that I wasn't trying to take them away from their religion. And that there was nothing about race that stopped them from being able to access such an important tool and technology. While I was teaching people of my generation, I couldn't break through. It just wasn't happening literally for decades, even though I was doing a lot of work with people living with HIV positive.

And, in fact, the African spirituality, which is incredibly close to the yoga spirituality, was quite oppressed and very much colonized.

So around 2015 I gathered a group of young people up to their mid-30s, starting from late teens, who were really keen to be able to work with me and to be trained by me. And it became very clear during the time that I wasn't reaching some people; I needed to train others because my reach was just too small. And obviously I'm one person. So in 2015 we started an organization called Kundalini Africa Rising and I began training teachers of color. Up to that point, there were no teachers of color teaching in the field that I teach in, which is Kundalini yoga. And then I developed a form in the intervening years before I started Kundalini Africa Rising. I developed a form which combines the two philosophies as much as they do overlap.

I use both systems. I don't use the practices because I've developed different ways of working. It's become a very popular form in a small way. It appeals to the African understanding of spirituality and it combines the incredible physical and mental practices that come out of the yoga teachings that we all know about.

The youth were really wanting to be trained as therapists. The reason why I went into training in the first place was to promote understanding in our national health system. In fact, the African public health system now knows how important it is to bring yoga therapy into public health settings.

The work is an amalgamation of two ancient indigenous knowledge systems. I haven't really created anything. What I've done is to draw from different philosophies and practices and put them into a form which is extraordinarily effective, especially here in Africa. For the reason that you talked about overlapping circles, I recognize the ancestors as a very, very important part of who we are. It comes from my own tradition where the ancestors in my culture are incredibly important. We keep them with us all the time. We refer to them all the time as if they're still alive. We speak to them. We ask for guidance. And so that has been a natural point of connection with the African healing system, which sees us as being part of a far larger system which spreads across different parallel realms.

So that is the one system. The other system, as you mentioned, is the earth and the land. I called it the earth because land has connotations of colonization. The earth bodies, the mountains, the rivers, the trees; they inform us all the time that as long as we are incorporating that expanded presence within, so we can really access those larger systems of wisdom inside of our own bodies. There's no difference.

In the teachings in Africa, you can't separate yourself from the earth bodies. And in yoga, it's the same thing. We are made up of these elements. We're made up of the same elements that are found everywhere else. So the practice is really being able to incorporate that into every moment, into every thought, into every relationship that we have with each other so that we are never just operating from that finite self, from the ego self that is always coming with these massive systems of energy that we're all part of together.

We are an organization that promotes actions. So we do protest marches. We're yogis, so we do them chanting. We're sitting in meditation, but we've got the placards and we've got the signage. And we are very clearly standing for a particular way of being in the world. So Black Lives Matter is an incredibly important concept for us and to see the U.S. rising and creating conscious awareness of what a scourge that type of racism is. It is a false category that makes people into economic objects that can be exploited. And that's what we stand for. We stand for a conscious awareness that we will do everything that we are planning. We used to be locked down here, but we are planning a silent protest march. We'll stand two meters apart with our masks on, and we will stand outside the U.S. embassy on June 16th, which is Tuesday—a very important day in history in South Africa.

We transcend the physically distanced through the heart space. So for me it feels very important and very relevant to locate within the heart space and then to feel the navel, the belly and the will, and to feel how that connects with our hands and how we translate that. And we manifest. You called it crystallizing. We manifest out in the world to the externalization of the self. What comes out of that when it's totally open and spacious is certainly out of our control, but is very magical. I love how we're embodying that space together right now. We're actually creating something magical right now.

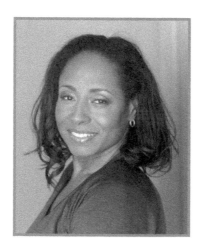

• • ● • •

Amina Naru, past Executive Director of the Yoga Service Council, is the owner of Posh Yoga LLC in Wilmington, Delaware, Co-founder of Retreat to Spirit, an active member of the board of directors for the Accessible Yoga Association, and works as a trauma-sensitive yoga teacher, wellness educator and workshop facilitator. Amina is a contributing author to *Best Practices for Yoga with Veterans* (YSC/Omega, 2016) and *Best Practices for Yoga in the Criminal Justice System* (YSC/Omega, 2017). Amina has been featured in *Yoga Journal*, *Yoga Therapy Today* and on the J. Brown and Yoga Alliance podcasts. She served as Executive Director of the nonprofit Empowered Community and is the first black woman to implement curriculum-based yoga and mindfulness programs for juvenile detention centers in the state of Delaware.

Amina Naru

Let yourself be your own guru, your own teacher. We can take the Buddha's story and we can take Jesus. These are external things. When you have it here within yourself to access, we can use those stories as examples and those teachings as examples to help inform us, to get to the realness of the lived experience right now.

What I do individually is work in the community through my business called Posh Yoga, which is bringing trauma-sensitive classes to juvenile detention centers and adult prisons. I also work on collaborative projects that I'm doing with Retreat to Spirit or with Pamela Stokes Eggleston.

I met Pam at a Yoga Service Council conference. We talked, we kept in touch, and I guess it was almost two years, three years later, we were on the board together. So from that initiation of connection and knowing that we work very well together, we have come together to combine our skills and experiences to create something that is larger and bigger than us, that we feel can benefit and help advance society. People who are looking for tools and a way to navigate life and the realities of life. People who are coming from backgrounds such as my own, and who are living in communities that I serve.

I'm speaking to all of the many projects that are within our co-leadership project.

After our tenure with Yoga Service Council ended, we realized people were coming to us and saying that they want to help. "We want to be a part of whatever you're doing. Talk to us, let us know what your next steps are. Let me know how I can assist."

We had Retreat to Spirit already set up. The feedback that we got from the people who wanted to help us was: "We've been watching. We've seen how you work, we like your co-leadership model, and we see the work and the impact that you two working together has had on the community, the yoga community." So it was more of the folks coming into us and saying, "Use me however you want. Let me know what's happening and how we can help."

I think my own personal practice of meditation plays a heavy role in this. Like the rooting part of my self-inquiry, and holding myself accountable, the end of the night checklist of what I could have done better, how I could have showed up differently, what was brave. Using all of that as inventory to inform how I show up and do the work that I do. So it is the conscious relationship with myself that I would hold paramount to feeding how I show up.

Also, in that comes the connection to spirit, so that's my ancestors, that's my spirit guide, that's the spirit realm that I tap into on a daily basis for support, for conscious awareness, to stay grounded, to receive information. I feel there's a third thing I want to say, but that's my top two. I am rooted in my practices of meditation, which help me to have that conscious relationship with myself, so I can show up and have conscious relationships with others. Then my strong support system from spirit, and then the third piece would be my support system from mentors, people who are helping us in our business, as well as personal mentors who are outside of my yoga community who have had the history with me as a friend to be able to guide me and let me know my goal points and where I'm coming from, versus where I am now.

How the guidance comes into me is textural. I try to explain this to some folks, but when I start to explain it, I judge it as like, "That doesn't sound... Do you understand what I'm saying?" You know what I mean? So I will attempt to explain how the messages come, because it is visceral, it's felt, it's something that I feel enter my body. So it comes in as a texture, but not as a tactile texture, not like something I can physically touch, but a texture as in vibration. This vibration feels soft or this vibration feels like trauma, this vibration feels like abuse, this vibration feels like love and support and understanding.

So the messages from spirit and universe come into me as textures, which penetrate my emotional body, and that's where it gets translated. So the translation happens through my emotional body, my heart, spirit, and then I'm able to understand the language, like what is being given. Then I process it to be whatever I need it to be, like, "Okay, I got that. Thank you. Now I know what my next step should be or how I should proceed."

So this relationship of co-leadership has often felt like a marriage, because I have been married before for 17 years, which gives me a texture to be able to access when I am interacting in my relationship with Pam. But what I have learned from that texture of marriage is individuality, so going into this leadership relationship with Pam allows me to practice that in a healthy way, which I didn't have the tools to do in that marriage.

Further, my meditation and yoga practice got me to being more connected to myself, so I know when to pull back and allow Pam to be forward and give the platform and support for her to feel empowered in our connection. It's mutual actually, so I think we model this for each other. There are times when I will feel very strongly about something and perhaps we're reaching a disagreement, but we're able to pull back and just agree to disagree. "I see it this way, and you see it that way. Let's sleep on it, touch back in tomorrow, talk about it again, see if anything else comes out of it."

One of the beautiful things about our connection is that we can pull from our tools, we can say, "I need a timeout. I need a couple days." You know what I mean? And don't hear from each other for a couple days, and then the other person will say, "Hey, is everything good? Can we talk?" And we're able to do that, and we're able to come back and show up and be present, and express and be vulnerable and transparent with each other, and offer that support for wherever we are in our personal life, as well as our professional relationship with each other. I'm not sure if I have answered the question, but that is what I feel when I'm talking about Pam and I, our relationship and some of the things that have come up for us.

Empathy, compassion, willingness to understand are leadership qualities I try to embody. Most important is co-creating safe space. If I did not have the internal space that I've created through my practices, I would not be able to hold space or be present for others. Not just my co-leader, but society, my family. So I want to say love, but there's this little, it's a little wavering when I say love, but there's some conditions around that part of it, I guess. But the love for myself helps me to be able to show up and express or hold love for others.

I feel like it's not the English language that I'm hearing from you to process; I'm processing feeling or texture. I hear the words, but how it's coming in is not words. So my mental mind is like I'm not answering the questions, but in my body, I feel like I'm rendering what is being asked. So for what you just said, what came up for me is, and we're talking about the root during my practice, there were many layers, there were many layers of myself that I had to uncover and peel back, that happened through my practice. Did I know that's what was going to happen? No, but as I practice year after year, month after month, retreat after retreat, these things just started to peel away.

The physical expression would be tears, gut-wrenching pain, like physical pain inside of my belly, things that were being released. I've been practicing this yoga meditation for over ten years now, and that is the root. I was peeling back, looking back on the practice, the layers were coming off, layers were coming off to get to the root, into the knowing of who I am, the knowing of what I am, and continuing to use that knowing as a source of energy to show up for others. I went way beyond a personality and what comes into the room. No, I'm showing up with these roots that I discovered through painstaking processes and tapping into that on a daily basis as my renewal to come back out into the world and society.

I don't have any stories or prepared teachings. I went through my 500-hour yoga teacher training, I had an experience with the Bhagavad Gita, and the Buddhist stories and religious texts, the Bible, the Quran, all these things I have pulled into my being just for intellectual purposes. But when it comes to teaching, I prefer to teach from my own experiences in life. I have a couple of sayings or quotes that I just stand by, and it's part of my classes. One is you can't see the picture if you're in the frame. That is my reminder to pull back, pull back, like get out of the picture. Like you're too tactile, you're all in there.

Of course, you're upset, you're feeling triggered, you're feeling this and that, because you're in it. Come back out, view it and gather the information and decide, ask for assistance and decide how to move forward. Another one of my most favored quotes is in the Serenity Prayer: "Grant me the serenity to accept the things that I cannot change." I struggled a lot of years in my life trying to control everything, being a survivor of childhood sexual trauma, but not knowing at the time why in my adulthood I had to have control over everything.

But taking the time to do some self-inquiry and read some books and tap into metaphysics and all these ancient texts, I help myself understand where that control or need to control came from. Also, anger issues and where that was rooted and stemming from.

I see and I feel that I see people being connected through their heart spaces, so there was a practice that you led us through at the SYTAR IAYT [Symposium on Yoga Therapy and Research sponsored by the International Association of Yoga Therapists] presentation when we first met, Allie, and that was the physical response. Put your hand on the person's back and then we turned around. I viscerally felt that, but the thought or the sight is what comes up now—the sight, the actual visual of that light. Which is this area, this space, this warmth, this light coming out as a cord and connecting to the next person and the next person, and the next person, and the next person.

So through the work that I'm doing, I'm just helping other folks to see that light, that ball of light that's there. They will recognize it, feel it, sense it, and then connect to the next person's light. It will just continue to go on like candles lighting each other. That's what I see happening, that's what I feel my work is, my mission is for being here on earth at this time, in this body.

If I'm not working towards that, then I feel I'm just taking my life for granted.

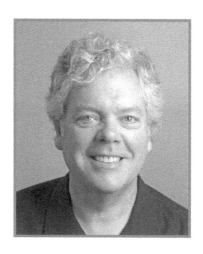

• ○ ● ● ○ •

Matthew J. Taylor has been leading integrative rehabilitation for 39 years and is the editor of the graduate textbook *Fostering Creativity in Rehabilitation*. He is a past president of the board of directors of the International Association of Yoga Therapists (IAYT), has planned many of their annual Symposiums on Yoga Therapy and Research, and teaches and consults nationally on business development for yoga therapists. Matt is on the IAYT PubMed-indexed *International Journal of Yoga Therapy* editorial board. He represents yoga therapy in integrative pain care and addiction policy development on national interprofessional taskforces, as well as IAYT's interprofessional collaboration business development projects.

Matt authored a book for yoga professionals titled *Yoga Therapy as a Creative Response to Pain*. He is presently engaged in a joint venture with a major health insurance company to integrate yoga therapy into healthcare. As a veteran, he's especially excited about initiating interaction with the U.S. Department of Veterans Affairs, assisting in facilitating how yoga therapists can be safely integrated into their initiatives.

Matthew J. Taylor

We take all this so seriously. And it is, but it isn't. It's like, how I am going to get through this? I don't think it's going to be the evocation and the making-things-happen kind of thing. It's the delight, the giggles, it's the being-mischievous kind of thing; later, when I was learning that embodying ways to learn to let go was a new path, I almost immediately felt my back open up.

I was working with people with 90 percent burns, and asking the question, "Where is the spirit to live?"

I guess that's what gave me a frame of reference.

I was doing all this innovative stuff that I never imagined myself to do. And I would go to all these courses and people would ask questions and I would go up and talk to leaders. I never thought I shouldn't bother them.

And at the same time, my lower back was falling apart.

What I discovered when I was exposed to the yoga philosophy was that, oh, all along I don't know where that came from, being left-handed, I don't know what it is. But I would listen, and I would support the whole person. I would remember Millie's cat's name. I would teach Mrs. Gurney how to breathe with her husband as she said the rosary with him as he was dying. It just made sense. It wasn't doing the technique or whatever.

But out of that, as I saw the model and the framework of the yoga, I was like "Oh, okay. I was dealing with this Kosha, that Kosha." And then linking back to that embodied sense of the breath and how that made safety and security for me and for people, and so my own physical practice of the yoga was pretty standard at that point.

I took a lot of asana movement, pranayama and Iyengar-oriented teacher training at the time as my entryway. But very quickly, I glimpsed around and said, "Oh, there's all this and it matches what back then were the beginnings of biopsychosocial spiritual practice as the groundings of traditional medicine."

I guess that's my dharma—to see connections between the two. I could see, "Oh, that's what we're talking about. We're just rediscovering it now. We're being able to see those cycles." As a recovering valedictorian, my way of staying safe is to get an A and to know stuff. I'm very much of an information gatherer. That's what I do, and then weave it and then tell a story about it.

And so that creativity, then, is that balance of action and acceptance.

That's what Krishna told Arjuna: "Shoot the damn arrow. I've got the rest of it." So we have to have both aspects. That just keeps happening on lots of different levels that way.

I think it's that safety and giving away what was coming forward versus holding tight to my vest. People say, "You're going to give me that?" And I'd say, "Sure, just do something good with it."

You need to understand money, you need to understand politics, you need to understand politics on a board of directors.

So my support came from having a kind of mastermind group or a community a little larger than just my one close confidante and being willing to learn and at the same time challenge them.

And I learned from an important mentor never to surrender my authority. Do not give over my place in the world even though I might be wrong sometimes. It was impressed on me that I've got something to do and I need to step up and do it. It's that willingness and that curiosity that binds us as *Homo sapiens* that hopefully we haven't had it squelched or stepped on along the way.

And so much of this may sound magical, and I guess magical in the sense of not being easily explained by current perspective versus the hocus-pocus and different levels of consciousness.

But these little sparks keep generating new opportunities and trying to answer my question, what happened in that yoga class. How could I, the "expert," not be able to take care of myself?

And what's the explanation? I ended up getting my PhD from California Institute of Integral Studies which is grounded in integral yoga philosophy. It was 2001 and that was when the whole yoga boom was happening, yet more towards the commodification of yoga. And I land in this program that says, "Oh, we don't do our practice for our enlightenment, we do it to raise the whole boat. This is why we practice." And that's the pedagogy of the school. So I get indoctrinated into that process, go through it and in that, looking at my own healing journey up to then and feeling and sensing what that was and how it could change.

I think, I feel, and I am a bit of a smart ass. I always have been. It's my sense of humor. I titled the first chapter of my book, "You Don't Understand Yoga." It's like everybody's writing these damn books as if they know what they're talking about. It's like I don't. I don't think you do either. And so, then I watched the clamor as the virus set in.

Everybody's doing asana practices and videos and it's just like, "No, no, that's not what we're being called to do. You're trying to have us do what we were doing, and it got us to do this."

And that's just back to my back. I was doing all these things that I knew to do that would just give me more back pain.

Maybe we go to the word mystery or the beyond-ness of the whole thing, of life that is magnificent and terrifying. It's both that and the virus doesn't give one crap about us. I think that's the equalizer that it is. So that humility of, we just don't know, yet there's this invitation to be surprised.

And so, interestingly, in just saying this right now, it's coming together as a realization for me that I love the craft of words and story and writing. So that now became a vehicle where not only could I tell a story, but I could communicate a story.

I didn't realize I was going to do it and I didn't have this proposal in the book, but my book ends up having a vignette of the epitome of my bad back pain where I'm flat on my back in a cabin in the north woods of Minnesota. One, it humbled me because I was under the impression that I had been trained to get just enough knowledge. Line up the parts right and you can manipulate the clock and get the clock to do what you want it to do. So there was a dose of humility with that and it was also embarrassing that I was barely able to kneel down and bend somebody's knee when my back is killing me.

They say, "Are you okay?" Oh yeah, just hold still. That kind of thing and what I've come to figure out is the yoga practice taught me how to be what I was saying. So at that time, I was saying I was a good Catholic boy and God would take care of me and I was safe. And then I was striving and pushing and holding and bracing like I didn't trust anything, and I was uttering from that standpoint.

When I was learning that embodying ways to learn to let go was a new path, I almost immediately felt my back open up. That brought ease and comfort, yet it also brought safety. In that safety and ease, I then found the ability to see differently. It was all meant to break down those walls. I think the back pain literally laid me flat, looking at the two and half pounds of drywall nailed into the ceiling in the cabin and counting every nail. It's like, there's something going on here and I don't know what it is and surrendering to that. So that part of the yoga, the last Niyama, just surrender to whatever that mysterious thing is. And that really brought me forward.

And to be okay with that and keep backing away and going to silence a little bit and then trusting what comes forward.

This time has never existed before. We've got to trust each other, we've got to be honest in our communication, and we've got to understand that we're going to screw up but we're also going to move things. It's never been done before. And we have to be supportive and as good or bad as artificial intelligence. If we move the needle and change things, this is going to scale literally around the world. You have many million beneficiaries around the world. So coming out of a meeting with a large healthcare insurer yesterday, I was just like, "Whoa, okay. This is where I'm sitting today," and now I get to have this wonderful conversation with you.

And I think that's what COVID is inviting us to acknowledge. This little, dinky microscopic virus that can get through almost any fabric is knocking us down and has literally slowed the world. Literally, and luckily, Netflix isn't infinite, so at some point people should run out of stuff to watch. And maybe we'll all sit down and shut up for a little bit and sense and feel.

And as you know, that's the magic potion.

Listen, something's calling us. Listen, listen, we can only do that initially by making space and being still.

There wasn't any sense of that laughing kind of nature. But now it's more a sense of me on my grandfather's lap and both of us chuckling because we just got Grandma to yell over to us, saying, behave or to settle down or whatever. And so when you ask what's going to carry me through or what that embodied sense is, it was lower than the heart, somewhere in here. It was just this unbridled chuckle, a giggle belly laugh.

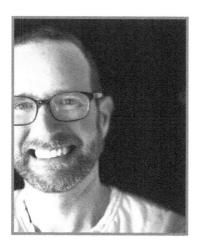

• • • • •

Jivana Heyman is the founder and director of Accessible Yoga, an international nonprofit organization dedicated to increasing access to the yoga teachings. He's the author of the book *Accessible Yoga: Poses and Practices for Every Body* (Shambhala Publications, 2019). He lives with his husband and two children in Santa Barbara, California. Jivana coined the phrase "Accessible Yoga" over ten years ago, and it has now become the standard appellation for a large cross-section of the immense yoga world. He brought the Accessible Yoga community together for the first time in 2015 for the Accessible Yoga Conference, which has gone on to become a focal point for this movement.

Over the past 25 years, Jivana has led countless yoga teacher training programs around the world, and dedicates his time to supporting yoga teachers who are working to serve communities that are under-represented in traditional yoga spaces.

Jivana Heyman

It just took a while, I think in my own maturity, in my own spiritual practice, to evolve enough beyond just yelling at people to feel that there was something I could do that's more productive. Yoga became the medium and the focus of my service. I could share yoga with my community rather than just be angry and sad about the people who were suffering and dying.

As a gay teenager, I felt separated from what culture was teaching me and I knew there had to be a different way. So I really started to look into deeper questions, especially because it was during the AIDS crisis and I had many friends who were sick and dying. And so I was really looking at illness and death by the time I was 17 or 18. These are already issues that I was facing and that I don't think most teenagers have to think about. So I was propelled to question the reality that most people accept and what culture gives out as the goals of life achievement—wealth and power and all those things.

I started to question all that early on. That's really what my work has been focused on.

Why do I feel motivated to serve in some way? I think I've always just had this desire to be used in the world and really committed to wanting to help remove the suffering of others. I've always felt that drive. It's just been in my consciousness since I was a child. My father was a photographer, a photojournalist, and traveled all over the world. I remember always looking at his photographs and thinking, I would really like to reach out to the world in the way he has. So I think he models for me. He just traveled so much, and I was really intrigued by that idea of connecting with people.

I was a visual artist. It's interesting you mentioned the visual because that was so important to me and that's what I studied in school. Painting and drawing were my whole life. Then there was a moment where I think I had a realization that it didn't feel like service enough to be creating art. I felt limited in some way that I didn't know if I could, in fact, be the change that I wanted to do, the service I wanted to offer in the world just through visual media actually. So I remember when I discovered yoga, which was when I was quite young. It had always been there.

My grandmother taught me yoga as well when I was a small child and then I came back to it right after college and it actually felt like a medium that I could work in more than just visual art. So yoga became to me a much deeper medium because it was spiritual; it was like the teachings and the practice and it was embodied in offering. It had so many layers of potential for me, for my own work and service, I think simultaneously. Instead of just painting, yoga actually has so much more depth.

I landed in a place, San Francisco, in the early nineties when AIDS was taking over. The government would not speak of it. There was so much homophobia and a lot of hatred and so that was clearly a place I could offer service. I was very drawn to that and started with activism. I was on the streets.

In 1995, I had actually been doing a mentorship with an individual teacher who was an incredible gift to me. I spent four years with her, a Japanese yoga teacher in Berkeley. She took me on as her apprentice and she was teaching me to cook and to garden and she was teaching me how to be a person. But I was frustrated. I wanted to go and serve. I left her after four years and went and took a regular teacher training program.

I started teaching in 1995. At the same time, my best friend died of AIDS. So it was a turning point year for me, where I realized I could use yoga to serve the community that I was committed to caring for.

Frustration is anger. We can go so easily there. It allows us to avoid so much, we avoid facing our own responsibility to actually create something.

There was a march on the streets of San Francisco. There was a group that we were protesting or something. There were two opposing groups and they had met up and there was so much anger there. You can imagine this yelling and screaming, a conservative religious group and then this activist group. I had been practicing for a while and I just had this kind of, I don't know, recoil feeling. I just had to get back, get away from that. I remember seeing these two men at the front screaming at each other on either side, the two different sides, yelling at each other, and they looked so similar. They were both angry and red and screaming.

I had this realization: this anger is only going to get you so far. This is not the way I need to be going. In fact, what I saw is that those two men were basically the same in their anger and they were stuck there.

And so I stopped. That was the end of my activism in that regard of being angry on the streets because it felt very limited. There's a place for it. I think demonstrating in a way is the grossest level for this kind of change to occur. We need civil disobedience. I feel strongly about that but there has to be deeper work done.

In chapter two of the Bhagavad Gita, Krishna is describing the problem, the human condition; basically, what we generally do. He's trying to show that you can live in another way: you can have a spiritual life. It's chapter two shloka 62 and 63. From brooding on sense objects, attachment to them arises. Other than attachment, personal desire is born, and from desire, anger appears. Anger confuses the thinking process, which in turn discerns memory and memory fails, reasoning is ruined, and when reason is gone, one is lost. But then you can go get disciplined in mind and have control of it. The sense can move about amidst sense objects, free of attraction and aversion, settling more deeply in tranquility, and in that tranquility, all sorrows fall away because the discerning is the effect of a calm mind is that it is tuned, secure and in equilibrium.

I do think that's where Accessible Yoga began. That's the main project I have. I realized that rather than protesting, I could do something more creative and service-full and that would be to share yoga with my community. I started teaching yoga for people with HIV and AIDS. I just put my energy there and it was really powerful and transformative for me. I found people were really thirsty for the teachings, especially people who were facing illness and disability and death; they became my teachers.

AIDS was barely treatable. There were very few medications. So many of my students died. I volunteered at an AIDS hospice and I got to work for people who were dying. It was very educational for me and opened my awareness more. I asked, "Having this limited time here and this body and mind, what do you do with that time? What can you do to make it worthwhile?"

Anyway, I started teaching a lot and those classes just kept expanding and I started including people with different disabilities, and Accessible Yoga was born from that—from that shift from angry and demonstrating to wanting to actually just share yoga with people, to support them, to give them access to the practices that were helping me.

I'm really intrigued by this idea of clear thinking versus egoism. I think that's what comes up for me: that question about ego and how much am I doing it for myself, while I'm actually doing it as a service to really focus on others. It's a blurred line because you can be serving yourself as you're taking care of others.

They go together, which I guess gets back to your point about the "*me*" and the "*we*." But I would say that I too often hear spiritual teachers use a lot of platitudes around the idea that we're all one, which is spiritual bypassing, and it's disregarding the challenges and suffering of people, especially those who've been marginalized. So I think it's really important to not just go to "We're all one" and to really look at how we're different. And the only way I can think of doing that personally is to constantly reflect on my own position, which is what you're asking me to do actually.

If I can be honest with myself about what I'm looking for, what I'm trying to get for my own needs, my ego and how it comes in, I think about how much more service I can offer. So I do that, rather than denying those things, which I think is how I actually feel. I've been trained in a sense to deny my needs and myself, my ego's needs. I actually think I've been very forward about them and being honest with myself about it is much more effective.

I'd say the next big leap for Accessible Yoga was about maybe eight years ago. I had moved away from where I'd been living for 30 years. I moved to Southern California and I left my yoga community and I was really struggling again the first time. It's always these struggles that helped me move in my life. I don't want to admit that but it's the big challenges that have offered huge benefits and rewards and that's what happened. I barely knew anyone. I didn't know anyone down here. Then I started to realize that other people almost feel the same way, that other yoga teachers, especially those who work in the area that I am interested in and that is bringing yoga to people that don't normally have access. We don't have a community; we don't have a support network.

I had this idea of supporting them in another way.

I realized that that jealousy, again, was my ego talking and how can I work with that and use yoga to really transform within myself that feeling of jealousy because I knew in my heart that that jealousy was for another teacher's success.

She was teaching yoga for people with cancer and I was jealous of that. And I thought, what is that? That's the most strange, this professional jealousy thing. But I was like, that's such a strange thing. I loved her. I love what she's doing. I want to celebrate her. My ego has turned it into some kind of a negative thing. And when I saw it clearly, in a glimpse I saw and what I realized was I needed to support her and I had this vision of her on a stage of, oh, I need to put her up on stage. I need to lift her up. And that was an opposition to what my ego wanted because my ego just wanted me to be lifted. And I said, no, no, it's not that. I love her work and I really do admire her so much.

That's how I had this idea of doing a conference, having an Accessible Yoga conference, and I did, I had her on stage and many others. I basically created a platform for the voice of the people whose work I admire and who I wanted to hear speaking. I created that platform myself and I was able to get out of my ego for even just the moment that some progress could occur.

III

Connecting to Source

Awakening into the Immanent,
the Emergent

Unfolding the "me" into the "we."

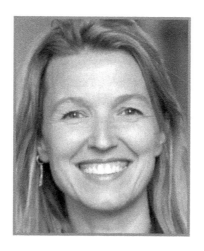

• • • • •

Anneke Sips is a community psychiatric nurse (RN), a Svastha Yoga Teacher Trainer (YACEP) and Therapist (C-IAYT) who has been working in the field of psychiatry since 1998. With her holistic and compassionate approach, she supports many clients in private sessions and group therapy. She is passionate about supporting others integrating yoga in their life and work, by leading the 200-hour Svastha Yoga Program for medical professionals. She is the founder of Network Yoga Therapy and the Yoga Therapy Conference in Amsterdam, the Netherlands, and a bridge-builder in the field of yoga therapy for mental health. She is a mother and enjoys her travels and dancing Hula.

Anneke Sips

And then I made it a consistent thing, a couple of times per year, and I kept doing it. I thought, after the tenth time, I thought, "It's nice to invite some guests as speaker, because there are all these researchers." I invited a few people, a researcher, a yoga therapist. They all said yes. So I said, "Okay, let's bring them all in." But then to bring all these people for 20 guests, that's weird. So then I started to invite more people in, and that was the first conference. The first International Conference of Yoga Therapy in the Netherlands.

It all started with recognizing curiosity and recognizing elements and characteristics in myself that people reacted to. I saw that I was doing certain things and people were reacting to that.

My dream was to create a multidisciplinary team and bring yoga into healthcare from the inside out. That is manifested now: I am teaching a 200-hour Svastha Yoga teacher training program to medical and health professionals! Followed by the Svastha Yoga therapy program! It's not only amazing to work together with Ganesh but also great to create this multidisciplinary team of professionals with one leg in yoga and one leg in healthcare!

And for other bridge-builders, I created the online membership called "The Bridge" that has the "Be Your Own Therapist" program in it with the goal of bringing like-minded community together to get inspired, learn and connect to the trend of the professional taking real good care of her- or himself by creating rituals for sustainable change on a personal and (since all is connected) global level.

And actually, now that I'm in my head, I'm back to when I was like 14, 13, like a really young age. And so I can say these are characteristics that belong to me. This is how I developed myself. How I was born, how I developed, the way I was raised, everything together. And it started to really express itself in that young age, the beginning of my teenager years, because I became more labeled because I was in a religious environment, especially my father—my mother not so much, but my father very much. And so the way I was being, my being was being labeled in a certain way. I was a Jehovah's Witness.

This was a little bit painful because I was wondering, I was asking questions. I was easily distracted; I always had a lot of friends. I was always the person who liked to play with the kids that were being bullied.

So taking care. I think I was caring, curious, outgoing, all over the place, not very concentrated, but moving through life like this.

I felt the impact because this was more on a personal level, like on the interpersonal level.

When I was 16, I had an accident and trauma happened where my liver broke. There was a lot of internal bleeding and because of the religion of my father, he said that I could not get a blood transfusion.

Well, this was a life-and-death situation. The doctors had to give me blood. So, they put me out of the responsibility of my parents through the court. They did give me blood but, of course, that was a big issue in the religious community.

There was a big milestone there in the development, but also that became a very important part of my development itself because after that I recovered. It took me like six months or something. And then I found out about that whole story and what happened exactly, and I decided I did not want to be part of the religion anymore.

I knew that if I was going to decide that, they would excommunicate me. I was still 16. I knew that if I chose to not be part of it anymore, I would lose my community there, including family, and that becomes very difficult. My mom was always supportive, but my father was very much in vain and he didn't know what to do.

And I think that all these qualities were really leading me. But at that time, I was too young, I didn't understand it. I had no clue where it all was going, but still, I left.

A lot of people could be stubborn, and I thought this was a negative label.

Later I could unlabel myself, thank God, and relabel myself as being creative and an explorer. This is how the Hawaiians were—they would never find the other islands if they would not explore.

Being in this story, being in this situation, being young with a conflict with a father, feeling also a little bit guilty for the suffering of my father and all that stuff continues still. I'm stubborn, whatever. I continued my way. I was 17, I was 18, and it didn't go so well between me and my father. I decided at 18 that I should move out. I moved to my own apartment. A couple of months later, my father died in a car accident. So we did not really talk about all that stuff and he died.

That opened a new door for me, which is very great, I think. It really gave me a lot of skills and tools that I transformed into really good things. Of course, the first years, first whatever, ten, 15 years, it was not very easy to find something in that element that is very useful, like how really to start to thrive from something this painful, this big.

But it happened. It was a tragic accident and at that moment I had stepped out of the religion. Then two years later, my father dies. I had to figure out how to deal with that by myself, because normally you have your parents or your religion or something...there's at least something. I felt like in this way, I had no ground under my feet. I could go back to religion and maybe I could find it there, but I didn't want it.

I decided to search. My searched started, then also my yoga practice started. I was 18 at the time, in a small town next to my small town. I read all the books I could find about yoga. Taoism, Buddhism, all kinds of things.

And, of course, I didn't finish these books because this is my personality. I would just start reading and searching. And I had always this very strong belief that I could make it, yet I don't know what I could make—it's that I will make it. And in the very worst-case scenario because I don't want to make these years look all very rosy. They were very soft, honestly, but I survived into these years. And for whatever reason, I always had in the back of my mind, in the worst-case scenario, if everything collapses, if nothing goes right, I can always just go to Hawaii.

So there was always a way out, you know what I mean?

At that same time, I started to really think about my future. I started yoga practice and my search, and I went to nursing school and I knew from day one, it will be psychiatry. I don't want to go to a general hospital.

I struggled a little bit. Sometimes I had to redo a class. It was not very easy. So I stepped in a level that was a little bit too low for me honestly, in nursing school, but I stepped in anyway and I grew in my work and in the situation.

That was another struggle.

I think also if speaking about what is my way of learning, I think I was always challenging myself a little bit and always stepping just a little bit across the edge. And not only in learning and in work situations, but I did this in many things in my life. I think it made me explore the world, explore myself, my relationships. I think all that stuff adds to who am I now and what type of yoga therapist and what type of mother and what type of human I am right now.

I was working in psychiatry. I was practicing yoga.

The first time that I started to talk about yoga at work, I was working on an observation and diagnosis. I asked the psychiatrist, "Let's do yoga. Let's just do it. I can teach."

She said no. I could not imagine why somebody would say no to something like this. I didn't know how to turn that no into a yes. I didn't know how to explain myself very well. So I decided I'm going to study more. Study yoga and study this world and see how I can bring things together. I think that's where this first seed was planted.

And then, meanwhile, I also traveled a lot because I just like to travel, discover new places. I wanted to go to Africa, and I found this project where there was a yoga project in Rwanda where people were working with yoga for women with trauma. I decided to go there for three months as a volunteer, teaching yoga. What I've seen there, what I experienced there was so much crazier than all I had seen in psychiatry so far. Trauma so deep and so complex, because there were also domestic violence groups next to the genocide survivor groups. It was insanely traumatized, the community there.

I saw that yoga helped them. When I came back, I was convinced. I put just a simple note on LinkedIn: "Anybody else here in the Netherlands interested in yoga and mental health care?" or something like that.

Some people reacted to that—mostly psychologists, I remember. I was just going to meet everybody, because everybody who had the same interests, I just wanted to meet them.

I was connecting and meeting, having lunches over and over. After a while, there were so many meetings that I said, "You know what? Let's just meet all together. Let's just meet, ten at a time."

We did, and I was organizing this little meeting, and I called it a network meeting. We got to stay somewhere for free and we would just meet there. I had no clue what we were doing, but we were learning. And there we were, all with the same interests. We all had the same feeling, but we didn't know really how to bring this together. It was really about merging together.

And then I said, "Okay, let's do this again. It's cool. So who's going to organize?" Everybody looks at me. So this is, I guess, a natural thing.

I was like, "Okay, I can do it one more time."

At the first Conference of Yoga Therapy in the Netherlands, 145 people were there—145 people in a church. I got all my friends from the medical field. And they just came for me; they had no idea that there was a group of volunteers. We were just friends and we were creating stuff. I made a logo and the name changed; now it's the Yoga Therapy Conference.

Let me think—was it 2014? Oh, 2015. Then 2015 was the first conference. But before that I already had met Ganesh Mohan, so this was also a big influence for me. Because I was always attracted to Krishnamacharya, but I was doing Ashtanga yoga. I was practicing in that area in the beginning. Super interested in the philosophy, but I never really got the connection that I needed and what I really was looking for. And when I met Ganesh, I was like, "Yeah, this is exactly what I was looking for." Such a smart and intelligent and simple way of bringing the science together with a super-deep yoga philosophy. No bullshit. The good stuff.

When I met Ganesh and he was exactly the link that I was working on, between yoga and healthcare; he's a doctor. He also helped me to find the words to bring this into healthcare and do all that. But then also I met his parents, A.G. Mohan and Indra Mohan. And also, it's just something about their nature that helped. I studied a lot and I was still studying and connecting a lot with them. And they really were so inspirational for me! Well, you can imagine from my youth—the father, the religion, the doctors or the healthcare system—there was always also a lot of this power structure that was very clear and very much there.

And I've been challenged also to find my way as an outspoken woman, finding my way in this system—all these systems, actually. In the religion of my childhood, I was the one who was speaking too loud, asking too many questions. Literally, people would say, "Can you just stop asking all these questions and just believe what I say?" I know this is so against everything. It's so against everything. But it kept going on, always a little bit like that.

And then I am the way I am. And also when I was working with Mohan G, like A.G. Mohan, one-on-one or, or in groups, but also one-on-one, I was asking a lot of questions. And he would always say, "Great, ask questions, the questions are very important." And I was like, "Oh my God, seriously?"

And so I feel that in the yoga, it's not just the teacher. I feel it's really a very in-depth knowledge that comes from a very long-standing practice.

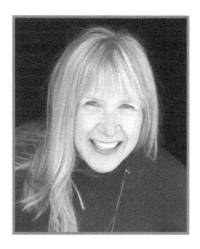

• • ● • •

Shelly Prosko is a physiotherapist, yoga therapist, author and educator dedicated to integrating yoga into rehabilitation care since 1998. She has a clinical practice in Alberta, Canada, provides continuing education courses for yoga and healthcare professionals, collaborates in research, shares her work at international yoga therapy and medical conferences, teaches in numerous yoga therapy and physiotherapy programs globally, mentors professionals, and is a pioneer of PhysioYoga. Shelly has co-authored several book chapters in yoga therapy and rehabilitation textbooks, and is co-editor of the book *Yoga and Science in Pain Care: Treating the Person in Pain*. She believes compassion, connection and sharing joy are foundational to healthcare.

Shelly Prosko

In this context, a tremendous trust emerged in the larger process, over and over and over again. Ishvara pranidhana. And that comes from deep within and has to be cultivated daily, of course. One of my practices is to first sit in a place of deep gratitude and feel it throughout my body. I ask for guidance and reflect on the feeling of letting go and surrendering to trust the process. I feel an embodied sense of allowing and trusting. It's not something I put into words, but a feeling I experience. And this also shows up for me as connection with others and the moment. One of my ongoing practices is to be fully present with the moment and anyone around.

What's arising now is connection to myself, connection to others and a sense of connection to something kind, loving and vast.

I remember a sense of urgency. I felt a sense of urgency to share these messages from the knowledge, experience and wisdom I had gained over the years. I felt a calling. I would be doing a disservice if I didn't share what I knew and had learned. I felt a deep courage and an undeniable sense of passion and conviction in moving forward. I'm not sure where this all came from. Even though I didn't have the language for that when I was younger, when I reflect back, that was always really important to me.

There's really no one particular moment or even specific driver per se. It's just something deep in me that made me understand that there is something more to this work. Something else that I think is worth mentioning is that I remember I started paying attention to times at work when I'd feel really alive and expansive. Those times when I'd feel like I was in the right place at the right time, doing the right thing, and feeling a sense of peace and flow.

And so that was early, early on in my career. And I guess one of the things that really inspired me was just recognizing that it felt right.

I started to learn about and practice other aspects of yoga, like breathing, meditation, awareness practices and some of the philosophy surrounding yoga. And I started to discover other benefits related to my mental, spiritual and social health. And when you have a daily yoga practice it becomes part of who you are and what guides you. You don't really take that yoga hat off anymore, no matter what role you are in, professionally or personally.

But as time progressed, and as the years progressed and I started integrating more and more, the clarity of the integration grew almost organically once I realized it was possible to do things in a different way. I needed to find courage to start having more difficult conversations and being more vulnerable, while still maintaining professionalism. It involved taking some risks and being willing to be unpopular in the mainstream traditional rehab setting. Of course, I wasn't the only one. It was a wonderful feeling to know that I wasn't alone, and we all had a support system.

I started meeting some of my colleagues; I recall so many conversations and correspondence among us. We all didn't really know what we were doing, and I'm not so sure we still know exactly what we're doing. But I do recall the increase of clarity to another level once I met fellow bridge-builders.

Like most things, the ability to offer that "something larger" and for a project to manifest, it often happens in small steps and takes a great deal of support along the way.

I remember feeling very alone with some of my ideas and feeling somewhat stuck for a long time. And then once I realized that there were other like-minded colleagues in similar situations, with similar interests and challenges, I felt more confidence and courage to be creative. It's like I needed to know I wasn't alone in order to give myself permission to forge ahead.

Many of the initial conversations and ideas about various projects began during those times, when we were all together in one place, sharing our experiences, stories and challenges. I attended IAYT's [International Association of Yoga Therapists] first Symposium on Yoga Therapy and Research in 2007. I met even more people. There were more of us that existed out there!

I felt like we were all sort of unsure and lost together, and trying to figure out things as a group. The Common Interest Community (CIC) sessions for rehab professionals led by Matthew Taylor was one of the things that brought us together to listen to each other's stories of what we were doing in our communities and start sharing ideas. We started creating a common language and building bridges.

I started sharing publicly about this integration and the work I was doing by speaking at the CICs, presenting at yoga therapy conferences like SYTAR [Symposium on Yoga Therapy and Research] and MISTY [Montreal International Symposium of Therapeutic Yoga], and writing articles for newspapers and magazines, including IAYT's membership publications. I think all of us bridge-builders who were doing these things were probably all inspiring one another to keep trying to forge a new path and to create various ways to share. And to this day, I believe we still do. And we continue to grow in numbers.

I was extremely fortunate to receive a great deal of autonomy and support. I had the freedom to try some different approaches in the traditional setting, but within the security of the traditional medical setting. I was allowed to offer yoga therapy in-services, write newspaper articles, change my service delivery model within the clinic to be more conducive to integrating yoga therapy, and was able to market from within the organization. I was grateful for that support and foundation and ability to practice and hone my craft and become more confident with this integrative rehab approach before I went out on my own.

I was delighted to meet another bridge-builder, Canadian Neal Pearson, from my same country. We were all carving a path together.

Our formal training program evolved. We had other licensed rehab professionals all learning together. It provided an opportunity for conversations and validation that what we were doing was actually a "Thing" we could name. It gave it life and gave us something tangible to hold on to, and even to have credentials and label it, I think, was helpful. I think it was an important step along the path to be able to have a label that offers some sort of identity.

It's been an ongoing journey of self-inquiry, discovery, acceptance and self-compassion. As I continue on the path of reflecting on my values and dharma, I try to make choices in favor of right action.

Sangha was and is so important. The external support, unconditional love and cheerleading from a small handful of people was and is so important for me. To see that others had the confidence in me and believed in me really helped me, especially through the tough parts; the courage emerged from that. Tapas is important too; the self-discipline to stay on track and not quit when it gets hard or scary is key. But self-discipline goes hand in hand with self-compassion. The discipline is easier to achieve if I'm truly practicing self-compassion.

Aparigraha has been extremely important on this journey. It's more challenging than we may think to detach or let go of the traditional biomedical approach and paradigm of thinking, especially when the common culture and majority of messages from authorities around us supports it and is so attached to it. So I've had to work at detaching from that engrained way of doing things and thinking to have the courage to be and do differently.

As I mentor those who want to embark on this path, probably one of the most common things that I hear from people who are starting out is that they find it challenging to take that leap into something that appears uncertain even if they feel drawn to it on a deeper level.

It's important to remind ourselves this is a normal and probably a very healthy reaction to uncertainty, and we can use many yoga practices and principles to help us work through the process and guide us on our path forward in a wise manner.

We have to start with cultivating the awareness piece.

I can see a future where we can all be even just a little bit more collectively aware. However, on the continuum of awareness, we're all at different levels of awareness. But even if that awareness continuum generally shifts us just a little bit forward, we all can be a bit more aware. We each start from wherever each of us finds ourselves. That will have a drastic effect on how we function physiologically as an individual and will therefore influence how we function as a collective.

If we can just shift that whole spectrum just a little bit more forward, I think that's the first step to improved health and wellbeing of the world.

Systems change is, of course, tremendously complex, and many factors are at play, but if we start with improving individual awareness, leading to a greater collective awareness, it could be a simple yet profound and powerful agent of change. It's the planted seed. When we look at yoga as skill in action and when we look at it from the perspective of gaining deeper insight into suffering so we can reduce or alleviate future suffering, we can see that awareness has an important role to play.

I can envision a future where we collectively have a better understanding and scientific support of the immense power and resiliency within living organisms, including humans and our environments. I think we will learn how to better harness the vital life force, particularly for healing, wellness and flourishing.

Currently, the health sciences are evolving to include mind–body–spiritual approaches in modern healthcare and research in academia, and the concept of non-dualism appears to be gaining further acceptance or at least some consideration.

Yoga therapists will be in a unique position, as we will be called upon to fill the gaps in the current healthcare model. I envision a future where there is a common understanding that we don't need external things done to us to be fixed, for the most part. The people we serve will understand we are their guides and facilitators of recovery and wellness, helping to unlock their body's own innate drive to heal, progress towards health and to thrive. I envision a future where we will integrate all koshas equally in healthcare, and where it will be commonplace to offer whole-person valued care that fosters connection, meaning, empathy and compassion in rehab and overall healthcare.

I believe the best way that we each can serve and create change is to stay connected within so we can be clear what our values are, and act in line with those values. We can remember that to serve self is to serve others, and to serve others is to serve self. That is one of my favorite mantras I use in practice. So, there's no separation.

We're really all one and in this together. Embodying this concept is what I believe is going to move us forward together and change the unhealthy systems, and help us grow and evolve as a species, as humanity. I think we also need to move forward with courage, humility and curiosity. Because this isn't going to work if there's arrogance, lack of curiosity, aversion or avoidance of uncertainty, and attachment. We have to stay curious, courageous, humble and be committed to service, and remind ourselves that service also includes self-care and self-compassion.

Lastly, I feel compelled to share something that I think we don't talk about in modern medical circles very much or at all, yet I think is so important, and that is love and compassion. I think we would all agree that these are important qualities of life and human flourishing.

However, we don't talk about them in the context of the interactions between health professionals and patients. And I think we need to.

We have growing research that shows the benefits of these qualities for mental, physical, emotional and social health, and we even have evidence that shows the benefits of compassion in chronic illness and chronic pain care for both the person in pain and the health provider or caregiver. And yoga therapy can offer a unique framework and offers many practices to enhance compassion and love, in ourselves and for others, and is inherently a loving practice where compassion emerges.

I can see a future where love and compassion are not seen as soft skills, but rather are seen as essential life skills that are non-negotiable in rehab and healthcare. I hope many will help bring this work to the forefront where it belongs.

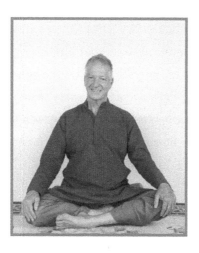

• • • • •

Joseph Le Page founded Integrative Yoga and Integrative Yoga Therapy in 1993, and is a pioneer in the field of yoga therapy training programs. He is co-founder and director of the Enchanted Mountain Yoga Center in Garopaba, Brazil, one of the largest yoga retreat centers in South America. Joseph began teaching yoga therapy in hospital settings in 1995 and continues up to the present as Director of the Healthy Heart Program, which conducts yoga therapy group programs in public health settings throughout Brazil.

He is the co-author of the book *Yoga Toolbox for Teacher and Students*, one of the most widely used materials in teacher training programs in the U.S. and in Brazil, published by Integrative Yoga. He is also co-author of the book *Mudras for Healing and Transformation*, also published by Integrative Yoga.

Joseph Le Page

What I feel is that all of us studying yoga at some level are gaining the qualities inherent in enlightenment.

Yoga therapy heals through education, through a group educational process. Tools and techniques support that, and, of course, research should support that. I think the confusion has come in, in that instead of developing what would be transformational models and then testing them, I think it's kind of coming backwards—where what's happened is we say whatever research proves, and that's the correct model.

As we move from "*me*" to "*we*," there are all of these different things. There are what the techniques do. There's the stress reduction. There's the psycho neuro-immunology, but then I think there's something higher. I think that the greater "*we*" naturally draws people toward healing. I think that that greater "*we*" is calling for all of us to be healed.

What do people need to learn about themselves and others in order to be healed? So that's the first thing. What kind of changes in vision and perception, in ways of looking at themselves and others in the world?

So that was the beginning of the learning, and then when we came to Brazil, there was really no yoga therapy to speak of in Brazil. I think we're still really the only ones. There are very few yoga therapy schools, but we started a program here in our local community, which has been running more than 15 years now. These people are fishermen. They're farmers. When you look at society and you talk about change in society, well, then you say, how are you going to change these people? How are you going to change the mass of the population who have these chronic illnesses? What we've found over these 15 years is that it really can be done. The way is through group support, through the sharing, through having a set of educational themes and having a sense of what perspectives, what new vision do you want them to have in each class? At the end of that class, not that they've done yoga postures, but that they've gained this new vision. At the end of the 12 weeks, they've gained a 12-part vision of a holistic self.

Then how do I take the yoga poses and make them support that vision? So every week the yoga poses progress, and every week there's an affirmation. Every week there's a new mudra. So how do I take those mudras and those affirmations and allow that to support that vision? Then how do I take the relaxation and make that part of that same vision? I take a meditation so that everything in that class supports that vision, so, at the end, I'm absolutely sure that those people really, as much as possible, have integrated and absorbed that vision.

There really were no other yoga therapy programs, except for ones in India, followers of Desikachar, whom I admire very much. I did a master's degree in teaching, and part of that was a thesis on student-centered learning. So everything that I had learned said that learning needed to be centered in the student. Then you take that and compare that against the Indian traditions, and there was just such a gulf there for me because everything there was different.

Even among the most open teachers, even I think they would acknowledge the best. Dr. Ananda—to me, he's the best. The whole society, the way of learning, it's very hierarchical.

In a certain way, I had to create my own methodology. It wasn't like I could choose between. There weren't any yoga therapy programs to choose from. In that sense you could say that, apart from Phoenix Rising, mine was the first founded by an American, and mine was the first in the sense of being yoga therapy in the traditional sense, covering what to do for certain health conditions.

I needed support, so my main supports at that point were Richard

Miller, I'm sure you know, and also Eleanor Criswell, the founder of somatics.

Of course, Richard and Larry Payne, the founder of the IAYT [International Association of Yoga Therapists], and then Eleanor who was on the board. I think she was president there for a long time. So they were the two that I chose, really, as my mentors at that point. It was a multi-year process that they were involved both as my mentors and as teachers in the program. So those were the two individuals that really, in a certain way, together with my intuition, created the Integrative Yoga Therapy program.

A couple of things that stand out for me was I remember Richard was a long-time student of Desikachar, and he had gone to do a research project there about what were the different protocols for these different health conditions. Then he found out that, for all the different conditions, the practices were almost all the same. So that brings in this question: Well, then what is the yoga therapy? How are people getting healed? Of course, the answer from the Desikachar perspective would be, "It's in the relationship with the yoga therapist."

But my focus was a little bit more on groups, on the social group, on the learning process. Right from the start, my question was: How are these people going to be healed? How does the healing process happen? One of the things I did very early was I participated for a while as a volunteer at Dean Ornish, together with Nischala Joy Devi, who was the head of that program. I was just a volunteer, but I did get to watch a lot.

I saw what happened in that Healthy Heart program was that it was actually the education that healed people. The group experience and the way that it's almost, you could say, a hundredth-monkey effect or the thousandth monkey or whatever you want to call it, so that people started to develop new perspectives. Then these perspectives came together in a group, and that's what led to change. Then there were these techniques that were actually just supporting that process.

That wave of knowledge was dictated by the five-kosha process. Then over time we could create the parallels between the five koshas and the seven chakras and the eight limbs of yoga, so really seeing yoga as one thing. So by taking that five-kosha process and organizing the weeks, this 12-week program along those five koshas.

I think that puts it in a nutshell—wisdom teachings in a convenient, accessible format.

Then you've got this other model, which is the research model, which is anything that shows research results in yoga therapy. In this process, what I would say is that the social change aspect, the change that happens in groups, the change that happens from perspectives, in people's perspectives on themselves and health, I would have to say that, from my experience, that part has been quite neglected in yoga therapy.

So in our case, we've been doing things like this Healthy Heart program more than 25 years. Our research was kind of cut short by the COVID, but now we're at a point where we can research. So I would say develop the whole methodology to ask: How are people healed by yoga? What is it that heals them? What are the different facets that heal them? So you have this facet of technique, which is important. The asanas do something.

So right away from the early years, I just dove into what would be the places where yoga would be least accessible to them. Senior centers. I started at California Pacific Medical Center, I think, in 1994. Then, in a certain way, experimenting. How do we make this process accessible to these people? I remember my first group of heart patients and just seeing what a tough nut a lot of these people are to crack and how resistant they are to change. I had, of course, all of these kind of Kripalu concepts, and I was a Kripalu yoga teacher. I still am in a certain way.

But I think that if we're looking at the future, I would say that my methodology is still to be recognized. It is quite contrasted with the current idea that you take someone and you do something to them and they get better. I would say that that still has a long way to go to evolve into something.

We've got the integration of 12 facets of a vision of wholeness. Each one is supported by a mudra. It's supported by an affirmation. We take that mudra and that affirmation all the way through the whole class. For example, our first class, I see the dawn of a new vision of health, and then we talk about how they see the vision of health. Then we bring that idea all the way from the affirmation. They create an affirmation. Even their breathing process, their pranayama, has to support that affirmation. Their relaxation, in the end, is where they actually visualize a sun rising, and it's a sun of health. It fills each part of their body. Then their meditation in the end is chanting their affirmation in a loud voice, in a medium voice, in a low voice, and then just listening to that affirmation internally.

So the whole class, this whole idea of a new dawn of health, it starts with an education. It goes to an exploration where they question themselves. What do they want to get out of the course? They talk to a partner, and then we bring that into the affirmation, into the mudra, into the asanas, into the relaxation, into the meditation. Then, at the very end of a class, each one shares one word of what their experience has been. They'll say things like "wholeness," "integration."

What it shows me is that if you have the right methodology, the whole of the population can be brought into these programs.

We'd been doing these Healthy Heart-like programs in the United States already for almost a decade. So when we moved to Brazil, it's just like this is what we do. We do these social yoga programs. Contacting people in our local community, they really had no concept at all. But they were willing to try, and we had this institute willing to finance it.

So what they found and what we found is that all of these social barriers, all of these cultural barriers, myself being a Brazilian American or an American Brazilian, having both nationalities, and that all of these barriers can be overcome.

What we're doing now is we're taking the 12 weeks of the Healthy Heart program and making them into a video program, a 12-week video program. So the classes will be shorter. They'll be 30, 40 minutes instead of an hour and a half. But what we would like ultimately is to see the Healthy Heart program in every community. Brazil is mostly public health. So we would like to make that available to public health throughout Brazil, either in the video format or when teachers are available. So that's our goal, and the goal is drastic and dramatic social change.

Even today I would say that communication skills, probably, in yoga therapy courses, is one of the things least covered. Probably the best in that would be Phoenix Rising founders, Michael Lee and Lori Bashour, in terms of teaching communication skills.

So what we found is that we could bridge all of this and that this is what these healthcare workers, the administrators, the nurses and the doctors want. They want their clients to feel at home. They want people to feel cared for. They want people to feel loved. They want people to feel included. They want to be sure that people are not being taken out of their depth. They're not being thrown into some weird spiritual water. That is actually quite a lot to put together in a public health setting.

So eventually someone's going to have to provide those means. And we're already starting to see that in public health here in Brazil. We are already starting to see that this is the only way things can work. This is the only way it can go, if people start to see the healing process as something more than taking pills.

I've been on this 15-year quest to understand the yoga sutras, and so I see everyone on this journey toward enlightenment. So if we look at the different words for enlightenment, I think each of them sheds light, so the first thing is that I need to go out beyond this personality. So I need to be autonomous within my true being so that all of this conditioning which keeps me from healing can be released. Then if we look at the idea in Vedanta, moksha literally means freedom. So within that freedom in Vedanta, I see that the *"me"* is *"we,"* a way of expressing that is quite different from yoga.

So for me, the absolute knowing, not a philosophical knowing or a theoretical knowing, but an absolute lived experience of who I am, why I'm here, is what my mission is. It's so clear, as if I'm looking at my hand and asking myself, "Is that my hand?" So it's that knowing. Then the other part of that would be limitlessness, that I'm not limited to this mind. I'm not limited to this body. The next quality would be wholeness, that there's nothing that I need to do. There's nothing that I need to prove, that everything that I need, I already possess completely and absolutely.

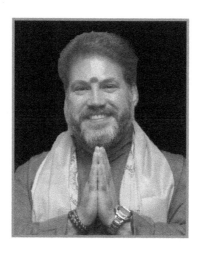

• • ● • •

Yogacharya Ananda Balayogi Bhavanani is the son of Yogamaharishi Dr. Swami Gitananda Giri Guru Maharaj and Yogacharini Kala-imamani Ammaji, Smt Meenakshi Devi Bhavanani. Ananda currently serves as Chairman of the International Centre for Yoga Education and Research at Ananda Ashram, Pondicherry, India, and Yoganjali Natyalayam, an institute of Yoga and Carnatic Music and Bharatan-atyam in Pondicherry.

He is Director of the Centre for Yoga Therapy Education and Research (CYTER), and Professor of Yoga Therapy at the Sri Balaji Vidyapeeth University, Pondicherry.

A Fellow of the Indian Academy of Yoga, he has authored 19 DVDs, 25 books and 31 compilations on yoga, as well as published more than 300 papers, compilations and abstracts on yoga and yoga research, and he is a frequent presenter at international conferences.

Ananda is an Honorary Advisor to the International Association of Yoga Therapists, Australasian Association of Yoga Therapists, World Yoga Foundation and Gitananda Yoga Associations worldwide.

Ananda Balayogi Bhavanani

What is a transformation? Everything we consider as normal has broken down. For all of us. Every part of the world. Now, the question is: Do we say everything is broken down, and break down further? Or do we say, well, it has broken down; what are the pieces I want to take out of my life and build the new that is going to manifest?

What is going to manifest will be a choice of what I am going to take from the past, bring into the present and help co-create a better future.

I consider to be born human one of the greatest blessings we can have, because to be born human is the culmination of many lifetimes of experiences, and the highlight of all those experiences, along with the karma that has been created. All this has brought us into the present form, where we integrated on this planet to work out the karma that has been accumulated. So, to be born human is a great blessing, and with the blessing comes a responsibility, and that responsibility is to live as a human being. Because to be born human, we are given a human responsibility, which is to manifest our humanity and grow into our divinity.

One blessing is to be born human; another is the family to which we are born, and my family into which I was born, consisting of my father and mother. Both of them, illustrious yogis, in the truest sense of that word. Both of them living a life of yoga in thought, word and being, and both of them on the path of conscious evolution towards the highest state of manifestation. My father had started the ashram in Pondicherry and my mother came all the way from Midwest USA to study with him, as a 24-year-old young American girl looking for the answers to the questions of life.

Marrying the swami... You can imagine when she took her husband the swami back to Midwest America in those days. And I was conceived in yoga. That is one of the greatest blessings! My mother, practicing yoga through the pregnancy, gave me a nine-month head start even before I took my first breath of life. So, when people ask me, Dr. Ananda, how long have you been in yoga, I say I have to give my age plus nine months.

Because it is not from my first breath of life; it was from the moment of conception I have been in that opportunity to live yoga as something that is every moment mindfulness.

Given the name Ananda, which means "joyful bliss," my father used to remind me... He said, "Ananda, when you do not manifest the joyful bliss in you and you do not enable others to manifest it through you, you are not living up to the name you have been given, and you have a responsibility to live up to that name of Ananda."

Yet when you are born unto this, the "we" is your natural state. And so, for me in the ashram, I don't think there was much of "me." The "me" moment, I think, would have been when finally, at the age of 13, I went to my first official school. And so I traveled. It was about ten hours away. About 300 miles away, in a boarding school in the hills.

I was on my own; I had to learn to take responsibility for what I was going to do that day. You know, everything starts to become a bit more of you, so I think that "me" point only started to come after about the age of 13, where I sort of was identified by me.

Because, up to that point, it was either I was part of the ashram, and it was more of being Samaj's and Imogen's son rather than Ananda. It was the school that gave me this "other" perspective, which then continued when I went into medical school, where, again, I went away from home. And so I was recognized for what I did, what I said and who I was, rather than he was so-and-so's son, or...?

So what is very important is not to rely on somebody else's answer, but to develop the capacity of self-reflection. And the way that can come into practice is breath awareness.

The breath is the key to coming into the present moment. There's no other way we can do it, to my knowledge. The breath, the moment you focus on your breath, you're in the now. There's no past tense, there's no future tense. You are in the present moment, the moment you focus on your breath. It doesn't matter what technique you do. Technique is secondary. People ask what technique? I answer, that is secondary.

Focus on the breath, because the breath is life. And where the mind goes, the energy flows, and the control of the mind is through the breath.

So the mind influences the breath, the breath influences the mind, and if you want to know yourself and find answers, you have to start focusing on your breath, not somebody else's breath.

My perspective on COVID is that it is the catalyst of transformation. It is not to be understood as an enemy. It is to be understood as a catalyst of transformation, because it is making all of us introspect. Every human being on this planet has been forced to introspect, and in many ways COVID has been the best yoga teacher. It has made people sit still, not go out, and to focus a bit more inward.

I respect all traditions because I personally believe every tradition is perfect within its own context. It is when we try to take it out of context that we end up in trouble, so this is a disclaimer type of statement I make. But in the traditions that I have inherited from my father, and he from his teachers, there is the traditional teaching. Yet because my father and I have both been medical doctors, trained in modern science, we have tried to express it in a way that the mind can understand and connect with in a more harmonious way, without diluting or distorting the traditional teaching.

So this is often very difficult, because when we try to take a traditional system and explain it in a modern context, one needs to understand both worlds. So the advantage to both my father and me has been that we were in yoga before we went into medical science. So we look at medical science through a yogic perspective, rather than looking at yoga through a medical, scientific perspective. And both are very different. So what we have is this concept that all practices are energy-based.

These are not just for the physical body, but we are an energy being, and I like to say that we are basically a big solar panel. That is why we need the sun. And our most important energy reservoir is the navel center.

So in most of the practices we give larger importance to the navel center, which in yoga would be called the manipura chakra, which is the energy that is considered to be of similar value. Yes, this is a traditional perspective, but this is, just as the mother and baby are connected by the physical umbilical cord, we are connected to the Universal Mother through the solar plexus.

So the manipura is our psychic umbilical cord to the Universal Mother, and when we are connected, we are healthy. When we are disconnected, we are unhealthy. It is as simple as that. So whenever we are doing the practices, the practices are all based on connecting and reconnecting to the source.

The main meal is the energy work.

And all the practices, when we do them, they are based on the concept of activation–deactivation.

We want a balanced autonomic nervous system, so that if you are in the middle of the road, and a truck is rushing toward you, you can just jump out of the way. That is what you need to do. But the parasympathetic gives you a life. So you need to stay alive, but you need to also have a life.

And that is why we start with sympathetic, followed by parasympathetic. Activation followed by deactivation. Do your best, leave the rest. That is what balance is. So every concept in yoga, every technique in yoga, is primarily aimed at enabling us to be a balanced human being.

Some of my students tell me I should have offered some sort of online programs, and everybody will be very happy. And yet one has to be careful not to get dragged into it.

It is a big danger. So, I think, keeping one's practice going, whatever one has evolved as a practice during this time to help us. How much of that can we carry into what we are creating as a new normal, so that the new normal doesn't reflect that old abnormal, which we thought was normal.

For me, it's like whenever they put out a new software 3.0; I like to look at this as an opportunity for humanity 2020 to be the best version of itself to date. This is how I envision and welcome this as a present omen of what could happen. That we have been given an opportunity right here, in our hands.

For humanity 2020 to be the best version so that, in time, history will look back and say those human beings on the planet in 2020 changed the course of human history.

I hope that will happen. I pray for that to happen.

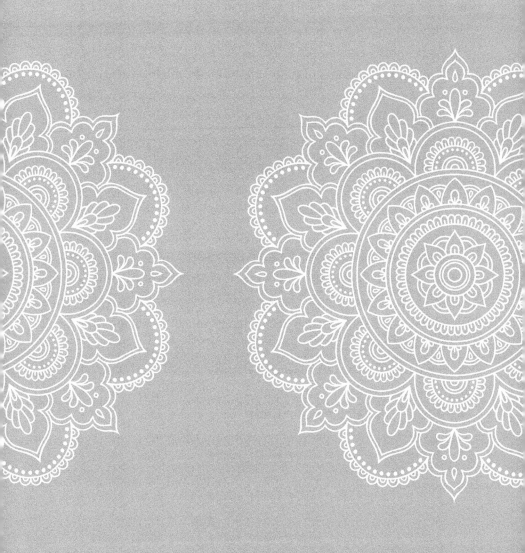

IV

State and Stage Shifts

Acting with Heart, Mind and Body as One

*Healing self and others by resting and
moving from a place of confident action.
Crystallizing, playing with a shared
coherent field of being-ness.*

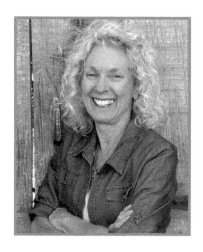

• • ● • •

Amy Weintraub was once an award-winning television producer suffering from depression. When she began to practice yoga, her writing aligned with her life's purpose. She collaborated with researchers and began to write articles and books, including *Yoga for Depression* (Harmony/Rodale) and *Yoga Skills for Therapists* (W.W. Norton). She founded the LifeForce Yoga Healing Institute®, which today serves students and clients and trains yoga and mental health professionals around the globe. Her *Yoga for Your Mood Deck* is forthcoming from Sounds True/Macmillan and her novel *Temple Dancer* (Tumamoc Press) has just been released.

Amy Weintraub

What's arising is my own personal mantra about being present. Our practices are there to give us compassion for ourselves, to bring a sense of connection to ourselves, to that which is divine within us, and to each other.

We are connecting through the one-on-one and the bigger "we." So finding a way every day to evoke that compassion for self that then expands into the "we," into the universe and for this planet of ours. For me, yoga, chanting—and I include in that chanting, pranayama, meditation, that's all yoga—is that portal into compassion.

Our practices are there to give us compassion for ourselves, to bring a sense of connection to ourselves, to that which is divine within us, and to each other.

I think that pain and suffering were the doorway, the portal into the exploration of yoga as a healing modality not only for myself but for those I serve. It was the rocky start that I had in life. It is in that dark night or that dark period of time that we can make a choice from and to that place. I discovered yoga and made the choice that this was going to be the path for me.

I would say the framework is deep pain that, for me, became suffering and then the release of suffering through practice and then the ability of developing ways in myself and others to ride the waves of pain so that they don't become suffering again.

I think that as I began to feel better and better, I wanted to learn what it was that was affecting me so deeply that I went from a place of deep emptiness—and not in a Buddhist sense of emptiness, yet empty—to a sense of fullness. What had made the difference? I knew at that point that I had begun practicing asana, pranayama and a little bit of meditation. I had a much too agitated mind to really focus and meditate at that point. I became passionate about understanding, so I became a Kripalu yoga teacher.

I began first to teach in my community and then I was fortunate enough that Rudy Pierce invited me to be one of the first outside teachers from the Kripalu ashram, which it was at the time, to come in and serve as a yoga teacher for a week or two so people could have time off.

I began this process of daily practice. I wrote an article for *Yoga Journal* about my own healing and did a lot of research. My article was called "Yoga, the Natural Prozac." It was the cover article in 1999, I believe, November. I think that's when it was. From that place, I felt like having done the research and having spoken to so many folks who could heal that it was now time to begin to move out with that. So my book *Yoga for Depression* came out of that. I had been teaching at Kripalu and I was asked if I would I put together a training. The book came out in 2004 and shortly after that I was asked to develop a training and I did.

That training evolved into the LifeForce Yoga practitioner training which is now much more robust and manualized for yoga teachers and yoga therapists and mental health professionals, as well as for other health professionals. It was kind of organic. It was an evolution from my passion to share what had transformed my life and to understand why it had transformed my life. I actually began to collaborate with researchers to document the changes and do research so that we could see what it was that was making such a difference.

I'm very grateful for people who were reaching out to say, "Thank you. This book changed my life." It wasn't the book. It was the inspiration in the book that brought people to the yoga mat.

What I was doing was synthesizing practices, making them

accessible to all folks, even in medical settings, who didn't want to practice yoga. I would be able to adapt and receive these teachings which I feel were life-changing, transformational.

I'd studied with many masters and I had integrated some of the practices that were the most healing for me and others. That, for some people, was not okay. It sparked a reaction of "How dare she teach aspects of this and aspects of that and she's not in a lineage? You need that lineage backup." Well, I had the lineage of Kripalu, but in some people's minds that wasn't a real lineage. There was that. I got in some hot water when I stepped out with my vision for integrating aspects of yoga from various traditions to support optimum mental health.

I should say this first: mental health professionals agreeing to train with me and become LifeForce Yoga practitioners had that sense of respect for the union of both mental health and yoga. I am not a licensed mental health professional but always had, even as a depressed fiction writer, that impulse to understand the psychological antecedents of why we do what we do and why we feel what we feel. It's always been a passion of mine.

When I started teaching LifeForce Yoga, the accepted practice was to teach energizing asanas such as sun salutations to folks suffering from depression and to teach calming practices for those suffering from anxiety (restorative, yin, etc.). While this is correct, I believed that those with depressed mood would be unlikely to be motivated, especially at home, to start with a stimulating practice, and those with anxious mood would have their rajas heightened if a calming practice was introduced too quickly. (I witnessed this repeatedly when asking agitated students to initiate Dirga three-part breath, to watch the breath, deepen the breath, or by asking them to begin in a restorative pose.)

My approach was to meet the depressed mood (tamas) with a slow practice that honored the current mood and energy, and then bring more life force into the mind and body by introducing more dynamic movements, tones and breath. On the other hand, if anxious mood is dominant (rajas), I recommended meeting that mood with a more dynamic practice and then, through guided attention to breath and body sensations, slowing the movements and breathing.

Meeting the mood rests on the principle of honoring the student's present state, without trying to fix it. Rather, we gently move into balance (satva) from either end of the spectrum. Meeting the mood was not the common practice when I started.

I had an experience in India long before all of this. This would have been in the early 1990s in which I had a teacher from the Advaita Vedanta tradition. I'm remembering a great poem of non-dualism essentially, Advaita Vedanta. It is said to have been "given" to Adi Shankara and is the foundation for Tantric (non-dual) devotional practices in the Advaita Vedanta tradition.

In this story, a little fish is out there looking for the great ocean, looking for God. "Little fish, just open your mouth, it's all around you. It's within you!" This story is like the universe is God and there's no separation, it's always all around us; essentially, that non-dual sense of Atman and Brahman as one. There was and is that.

I also know that chanting really lifts my spirit. Chanting evokes a place, or it brings me to a place that meditation also brings me to, not always, yet both meditation and chanting have the potential to clear the space, to remove the obstructions so that I reconnect with my own true nature.

Later in my journey, I read a quote from Swami Sivananda that validates the way in which I teach LifeForce Yoga: "Adapt, Adjust, Accommodate."

It was my own curiosity and passion to find out what it was that was making a difference. So I was a little bit of a nerd for a while. Now I'm just practicing and not as tuned in to the research. But for a while I would do at least a monthly newsletter. I would just stay on top of all the research that was coming out. When I wrote the book *Yoga for Depression*, there wasn't that much. I was going back to Shirley Telles and her really important work in the early 1990s on left and right nostril breathing. And then there were some works in the 1970s from France.

Yoga for Depression was published, and then more and more research started to emerge. I collaborated with some of the researchers but there was also a great flowering of research, this millennium—a great flowering of research. I just stayed on top of it because it would be so exciting to me to say, "Wow. This validates my felt experience. This study here on sound done in 2011 by the National Institutes of Mental Health and Neuroscience in India looked at om and found that it actually stimulated vagal nerve activity!" I would get so excited about what I was reading and, again, wanted to share it.

I remember when I started a program at the juvenile detention center here in Tucson. In my first time teaching these girls who had these labels on them of bad—totally not good enough but worse than not good enough, bad—I felt connected with them immediately. This was so inspiring to me. They came in. They were over-medicated, on a lot of products. They'd shuffle in. After the yoga class, there was such a transformation in their faces. They would share photographs and say, "This is my daughter, Missy. She's with my grandma."

I walked out into the parking lot and tears rolled down my face that this yoga could be so transformative. It was just a simple practice.

When people feel that this work has healed them and reached them and touched them, they want to help others with it.

They want to reach out. That's how I felt and that's how people who have read the book become yoga teachers, and then come to the LifeForce Yoga training. That's sort of the evolution of it.

You framed it in the beginning, this question of finding your true nature. That's the work for me, for LifeForce Yoga practitioners like you and others.

It's not about fixing or changing or having any agenda about what positive mental health is supposed to look like in the person or people you're working with. It is helping them clear their space, letting go of the story or letting go so their own true nature arises and they connect with that true nature.

It's all about co-creation. When I teach practitioners, it's also about learning the practices and making them your own. Make it work for you and for your clients. You know your clients. They know themselves better than you do, and you know them.

We can be inspired. We can practice. Relationship is the real healing element.

I can feel uplifted to a certain extent, but there's nothing like feeling community around you. Social distancing has limited that. I guess I am just looking forward to the time when we can gather again as a community in person because this time has its elements of disconnect even as we reach across the world to connect with each other.

But I think we need to go within and find the practices that we may already have.

Find the yoga teacher that inspires you, and if you're new to practice in these times, find it and just keep going back. Keep going back. Do your practice every day. Find a space in your apartment, your home, that you can go to.

Practicing in nature, whenever possible, means finding ways to live that place my hands in the soil, my face in the sun and my feet solidly on the earth.

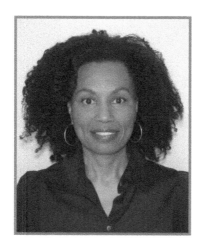

• • ● • •

Pamela Stokes Eggleston is the Founder and Director of Yoga2Sleep, Co-Founder of Retreat to Spirit and Adjunct Professor/Yoga Therapy Clinic Supervisor at the Maryland University of Integrative Health. She previously served as Co-Executive Director of the Yoga Service Council. She is a contributing editor of *Best Practices for Yoga with Veterans* (YSC/Omega, 2016) and *Yoga and Resilience: Empowering Practices for Survivors of Sexual Trauma* (Handspring, July 2020), as well as researcher/author of *Yoga Therapy as a Complementary Modality for Female Veteran Caregivers with Traumatic Stress: A Case Study* (Maryland University of Integrative Health, March 2018), and *Addressing Multiple Sclerosis Symptoms: A Yoga Therapy Case Study* (Maryland University of Integrative Health, June 2019). Pamela serves on the board of the international nonprofit Accessible Yoga.

Her work and writing have been featured in *Yoga Therapy Today*, Insight Timer, Meditation Studio, Gaiam, MilitaryFamilyLife. com, *Military Spouse Magazine*, *Yoga Journal*, *Mantra Yoga and Health*, *Essence*, *The Huffington Post*, and on *The Ellen DeGeneres Show* and MSNBC.

Pamela Stokes Eggleston

What's really important is soul care, spiritual care. Getting to those subtle energies and working with them. Really caring for them. And using the yamas and niyamas to practice ishvara pranidhana. That surrender to the divine and really working with that. What does that look like in your life? But the subtle energies, those energies that we learn about—chakras and nadis and all of these things that are really real. And that really live in our bodies, and they are our connection to our ancestors.

I feel like I have been surrounded by people in the space of yoga service, mentors, people that didn't know they were going to be my mentors. Folks that were working to help me without me asking.

I would say that this was probably about eight years ago. I was just interested in taking these different trainings through yoga. Trauma training specifically to work with veterans. I met a lot of great people, many of whom were veterans themselves who were working through their PTSD or their trauma with yoga.

That's how I met Rob Schware originally, because he was in DC at the time selling his house, moving to Colorado, where he is now. And all of these alignments happened without me really making a huge effort in that way.

So these people came into my life. People were like, "Hey, you should meet this person. You should meet this person. This person will help. That person will help." And the synchronicities that happened from that were amazing. I would get scholarships to trainings. I would stay free at places. I mean, it was amazing. Because at that point, I was a struggling yoga teacher.

It was just synchronicity. It was just an alignment.

Simultaneously, I had doors slammed in my face. There was this dichotomy of energy where I was getting a lot of support in one end and then there were a lot of people who were like, "We don't want you over here."

Because I got that support, the door slamming didn't dissuade me, right? I wasn't dissuaded by that.

With those two dichotomies, I learned how people move in this space. I was green. You think, "Oh, yoga, love and light. Everyone's going to be nice." I mean we know that people are people, but that was the crux of me starting to develop a particular style of leadership and mentorship in my own space for myself.

I had worked corporate prior to that. The universe says, "Hey, you should do this," and you do it. I had that type of leadership as a manager, project manager, assistant director, all of these titles. But the energy wasn't right. I left. I moved into this other space where the leadership seemed softer, kinder and something that I could accomplish more innately with the help of these different experiences. I won't label them good or bad. I'll just say very open, maybe not open, that cultivated a sense in me that was like this is what I'm feeling.

So, it wasn't an "Oh, I'm going to do this, I want to lead this organization or that organization." No, this was more about me being embodied in my practice through these learning experiences of doors being closed, doors being opened.

My husband is a wounded warrior. I shall begin that with the anchoring of when I started Yoga2Sleep. The impetus for that was my secondary PTSD, because my husband had PTSD and I sleep with him. I was sleep-deprived; it was very simple.

From that offshoot, I realized that many other people had PTSD. Veterans and the service members and the wounded warrior caregivers like myself who were taking care of them.

That was something that was organic and just became. Nobody

was specifically teaching wounded warrior veterans. Nobody was specifically doing therapeutic yoga with them. I've been doing that for five years with a nonprofit called Hope for the Warriors.

It was a calling to work with veterans. I started going to conferences at Omega with the Yoga Service Council. I started meeting a lot of people and we'd just see synchronicities that would happen because of the work that I had started doing. And then, subsequently, I got a contract. I'm a vendor for the Veterans Administration. The local VA here. And then, I started getting clients through that. So it was just an amazing journey that I was just getting put in front of these people and places and events, and just sharing from the heart what I was doing and people really resonating with it for the most part.

And the odd thing is there's a sense of worthiness. What is the worthiness that we have as yoga teachers, as yoga therapists to honor ourselves and honor the person or persons that we are serving in a way that matters? And by that it's not just money or whatever people know something. It's more like how are you really 100 percent showing up, honoring the people that you say, that you purport to serve? And are you an embodiment of that? That is my practice, to be embodied in that. And I know that we are not perfect, and we have our rough days. But that is the charge for me: to have a daily practice to always look at that. To always look at my stuff.

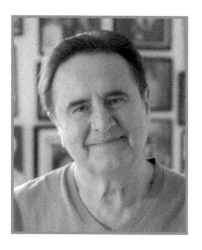

• • ● • •

Larry Payne is a yoga teacher and author/co-author of seven books. He is the founding president the International Association of Yoga Therapists (IAYT) and developed the Yoga curriculum at the UCLA School of Medicine. He is the founder of the Yoga Therapy Rx and Prime of Life Yoga programs at Loyola Marymount University, the corporate Yoga program at the J. Paul Getty Museum, and the original "Back Program" at Rancho La Puerta Fitness Spa.

Larry founded Samata International Yoga and Health Center in Los Angeles 1980, where he continues to teach groups and offer yoga therapy to individuals. A frequent invited presenter at international gatherings, Larry's most recent publication is the American Association of Retired Persons' *Yoga After 50 for Dummies.*

Larry Payne

Well, I think it's work to have a search. To spend the time and allow for the search. And for some people that happens; they're given it by their grandparents or something. But for all of us who've come into this path, there was usually this one time. And so I think it's about allowing yourself to have this search at and for the right time for you, and to follow your heart to where it takes you. And that's what I've done.

We were the ones that were like disciples, and now we're the elders.

So I feel pretty happy that I've taken it to where it is, and now I think I'm going to focus a little more on the category of yoga for people over 50.

I asked, "What is a thing that will help me the most to be a good yoga teacher?" And I was told, "Be an example." So that's what I've tried to do.

Okay, I was an advertising exec. And in that field the more you do, the more they give you. Until I developed a low back twitch. And as I look back on it, I think it was because I was sitting so much and working such long hours. And then they had a meeting for all the top producers, on an island. And when we got there, I noticed that every person in the group had a twitch. And they handed out these baseball bats that said, "Nice guys finish last," on a plaque. And that was the moment I said, "Get me out of here." And I came home, and I talked to my running partner about it. He said, "Why don't you come with me to the yoga class my wife goes to?" And it was a woman named Renee Taylor who was a disciple of Indra Devi. She actually met Indra Devi. So when I got there, she was old and kind and really watching people.

And at the end of that shavasana, when I opened my eyes, my back pain was gone, my twitches were gone, and I felt like I was smoking something. I was so high, and it lasted for four hours. That was the moment. And when I came home, I found a yoga teacher in my neighborhood because I had to travel far for that one. And I started taking classes and I didn't stop for the year. I gave notice at my employer and I took a sojourn around the world, diving into yoga and all of it.

I was almost 38. When I went to *McCall's Magazine*, where I was the West Coast manager of advertising sales and said, "I'm sorry, I quit," they were unbelieving. They said, "Don't quit, we'll give you a one-year sabbatical." So after I went on this trip I had no attachments. I was divorced, I had some money in the bank, I had a press card, I had a camera and a tape recorder.

So it came from a twitch in my eyes and a pain in my back like a dog bite.

Everywhere I went, people were very kind to me. And I did interviews. I started at a place called Findhorn, in Scotland. And then I went through Europe briefly, and then I just headed for India. When I got there, I knew. That's my place. I spent the rest of my six months in India and that's where I met all of these teachers. That's where I met Krishnamacharya, and Desikachar, Indra Devi, and all of these people.

The part I left out was that my local yoga teacher had these juice fasts on weekends. I enjoyed those. He said, "If you want to get the full benefit, you should do a two-week cleanse at a place called Meadowlark"—with a man there who was the father of holistic medicine in America; his name was Evarts Loomis. So when I went there, that was the final moment that inspired me to quit and to take this trip, or at least be on sabbatical. They would analyze your dreams and you'd journal all those things. So while I was there, in my journal I wrote down what I'd like to see happen. And that's when I took a trip to go find that. And he, Dr. Loomis, the father of holistic medicine, had taken a similar trip and he gave me names of people, in Europe especially, that he had met that I could talk to. And so I think that the vision still counts. If you have a spiral binder and you just put your ah-ha's in there, you don't have a method. So this was from 1998, and I put it in a PowerPoint just to show people. That's when it landed for me. And I wrote down that I went to this place that was for yoga and healing and international teachers, and that's what happened.

So I think I was lucky—being in the right place at the right time and having the background that I did.

The yamas are always pretty good, and so forth. I often go back to the yamas. So I think mine, it will not be something that's looked upon as the big intellectual path like a Gary Kraftsow or a Leslie Kaminoff or something like that. I'm more practical and down to earth, working with people. You know, if you're a new yoga teacher today, you can get yourself in a lot of trouble, if you have power, because power is something that really attracts people. And a number of my friends who were really good friends have gone down from that.

So I think that's something, especially as men, that we have to watch out for. To not let the power thing get to you. I always say that I'm a legend in my own mind. And I have a wife who reminds me that I put my pants on like everybody else every day.

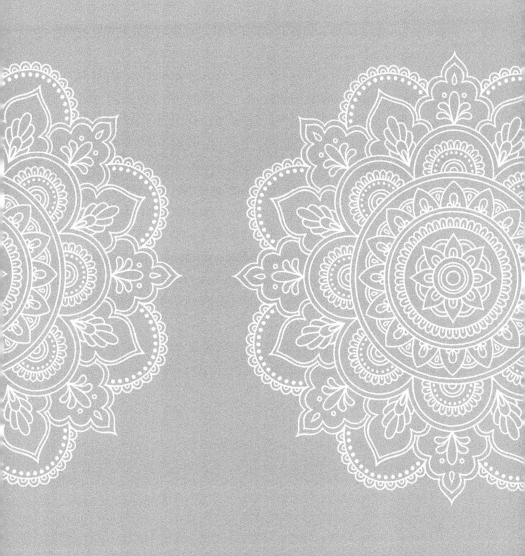

V

Transforming Actions

Conscious Engagement,
Stewarding "the New"

*Moving with the collective will as it
becomes visible, engaging with self
and others through all the senses.*

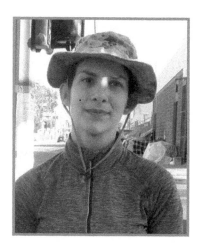

• • ● • •

Hi my name is Freidel. I am in the process of healing dissociative identity disorder. I am recovering from complex trauma that started from birth. I am healing from generations of incest and pedophilia. I am also healing from human and sex trafficking. I live with symptoms of hallucinations, delusions and other sensory perceptions which sometimes impact my wellbeing and functionality. I enjoy experiencing kindness and clarity, and I enjoy helping others in reducing suffering wherever possible. Growing clarity around the conditions that give rise to my own suffering allows me greater clarity into the conditions of other people's suffering. Specifically, I am drawn to focusing my mind on the continuum of causes giving rise to chronic homelessness, and to engaging beneficial action in protection of people separated from their own agency.

Freidel Kushman

It's about really meeting people as humans, and then seeing in clarity their circumstance and being able to reflect in clarity to them that they're someone, like me, who has an intention for well-being and has an intention for healing, health and overall benefit.

I live with a lot of hallucinations, and what I commonly refer to as mental health challenges that become the shape of hallucinations and voices. It's taken me a very long time to learn how to live with them, and to be functional in society with them. And I also come from a background with complex trauma from birth. So I feel that the way I exist in the world now has emerged from my own experience and suffering and witnessing the suffering in my environment. I seek the suspension of all suffering for myself, and for everyone connected.

I felt very compelled to spend my time in the Skid Row community here in Los Angeles. Skid Row here is called by some the nation's homeless capital. There are about 5000 people in the community. Most are black, most people live on the street. I felt very compelled to spend as much time there as I could. So I was just going there every day for five or six hours a day, and trying to make friends, and integrate into the community there at the street level. After some years of doing that, I think that people around me who were outside of the Skid Row community felt they wanted to be present for that suffering too in that helpful way.

Some of the primary features in the Skid Row community where I work are the impacts of systemic racism, the current and very alive manifestation of disregard for life. And systemic violence also, and kind of a preoccupation with personal comfort at the expense of another person's homeostasis.

I experience myself as working with everyone connected to me. I think there's a lot of people in local government there. There are a lot of people working with me and with my organization, a lot of people in residence just in the community, community residents and from other organizations. So I do experience myself as working with everyone in that way. Regarding the rendering of services, the organization and myself, we've gone through phases where in the first year of operating, rendering services was really just a group of us. I think there were four of us, three or four of us going into the Skid Row community every day for a year and a half and just integrating in the community. That time spent was the rendering of service. I don't like to say it that way because it was really an inner growth experience for me and for everyone. That is sometimes a very rare experience for people that have been chronically homeless. And then after a year and a half of just kind of doing this, then we started running pilot programs for about a year. And then we had another phase of only attending government meetings for about a year every day. And now we're in another phase now building out our pain care clinic. We've not rendered services yet because we're still building out the infrastructure. But that'll be coming in the next several months.

I think that it's possible that I have a different experience with yoga. Or maybe I talk about it differently than is common. My experience with yoga has been cultivating the ability to see myself and my circumstances and my surroundings in clarity. I think that having my own healing process from a lot of complex trauma, I am cultivating clarity by growing in comfort and to stick with my inner experiences. That's helped me to gain clarity. And then with that clarity, cultivating agency. For me, that's very much the yoga for me: having clarity about what's going on, about what's now, and then being capable to move in accordance with my own agency. That's very much my yoga.

I think agency is being who I want to be. In my life, I think there's been a lot of structural and other barriers that prevent me from being who I want to be. And I know the same is true for people experiencing homelessness. And not just homelessness, but people experiencing all of the social epidemics that result from systemic violence. So I know that's a shared experience: not having the resources, not having clarity and not having the relational support to be who you want to be.

I think we perceive that someone is choosing homelessness. That choice that we're perceiving was not a choice. And that resulted from or is continuing to result from an experience of structural violence or systemic violence. Whether it's harmful relationships within the new environment a person might be transitioning into, usually there's something harmful that someone is trying to avoid. And so being in a familiar territory, where one is familiar with how they're going to live their life, and how they're going to meet their needs is a much preferable option over experiencing a brand-new harmful circumstance.

There's certainly a lot to be said for communicating in government spaces from an intention to benefit others, all others. And speaking through a spiritual lens in government settings is necessary and naming harm in the moment is necessary. And every time that I've done that, or I've witnessed countless of my friends doing that, it's deeply beneficial for everyone involved.

Yoga, as I learned it and as it's been taught to me, has been largely inaccessible for me to practice because I don't know how to be safe, period! So I've been cultivating a practice this past year that is now my yoga practice. It's a combination of creating a safe inner space which is a space that I'm able to identify as somewhere that I feel protected. I have a lot of markers, different things that I use. I tour around the inner place, and I look at the markers because all the markers mean something different about truth and different realities and my reality.

Once I'm in that safe space and I've toured all the markers, then I have a tonglen practice of taking and giving. I sit in my clarity and

I investigate a site of my own injury, my own programming from my trauma history. And I see that in clarity and I move back and forth between experiencing the injury itself and then I experience the investigation of the injury. Then I practice compassion and sadness for the part of myself that is still experiencing that injury. And then I rinse that and I repeat that. And that's been my inner practice. I'm also adopting outer practices such as keeping hydrated and preparing food and practicing good hygiene, which has also historically been impossible for me. So, yeah, that's my practice now.

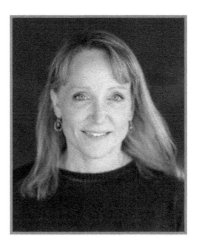

• • ● • •

Catherine Cook-Cottone is a licensed psychologist, registered yoga teacher and professor at the State University of New York (SUNY) at Buffalo. She is creator and director of the Mindful Counseling Advanced Certificate program and co-founder and president of Yogis in Service, Inc. a not-for-profit organization that creates access to yoga.

Catherine's research specializes in embodied self-regulation (i.e. yoga, mindfulness and mindful self-care) and psychosocial disorders (e.g. eating disorders, substance use and trauma). Her research has been funded by the National Science Foundation, UNICEF, lululemon athletica and the Give Back Yoga Foundation. Catherine has written eight books and more than 75 peer-reviewed articles and book chapters.

Catherine consults with the Africa Yoga project and the United Nations Foundation, to provide trauma-informed, mindfulness-based resilience training to yoga teachers in Kenya, Somalia and Rwanda, and humanitarian workers in North America, Africa and the Middle East. In 2018, she was awarded the American Psychological Association's Citizen Psychologist Presidential Citation.

Catherine Cook-Cottone

We ask: What is it that is happening? Is it the sensations, getting into the sensations of your body? Is it being so reconnected with your body, the proprioception, interoception? What is it that lets you reintegrate so that your intellectual self isn't running the show and you miss your life? Because essentially that's what can happen. We are all so highly rewarded for intellectualizing our way through the whole entire world and yet it's such an empty experience really.

I tried to over-understand everything to the point where it became not feasible anymore. Some things are not to be understood—they are to be experienced. And I became sick. I became ill with an eating disorder that I had for many years.

During that whole time, I also had a strong sense from the core of myself and my heart, that I was meant to do something with my life. Since I was very young, I had this sense I was here for a reason. I didn't know what it was. Without a reference or a way to understand this feeling, it confused me. I often didn't trust the feeling. So I would just often be sad about it when I felt it and confused by it and disregarded it. Not trusting any internal guidance, I would try to comply with external standards for beauty and performance. I did this for many years.

I wish I had a story that read like this: "I followed my heart from the time I was five because I listened to my heart and manifested my life from there." I have a picture of myself that I still keep on the desktop of my computer. My mother took the photo. It's me standing in tights with a tutu, with a big satin bow that my mom made me, for a little play we created for my first-grade class. I was going to be a ballet dancer in a skit with my friends. When I saw the photo, as a kid,

I hated myself, hated it. I didn't look like I was supposed to look. I was too round, too big. Now, I look at the photo and I just love that kid. I love how she wanted to dance, express herself, and she should have just been filled with joy.

Still to this day, that picture just breaks my heart in a really good way. I guess my heart needed to break. And so it's a bit of a reflective and generative story, as I now use the "little girl me" as a guidepost for my work now—the hope that kids growing up don't have the obstacles that I had. That they could just be in, of, and with their bodies. And when I say kids, I mean the vulnerable parts of self in all of us from zero to 100.

There's a child in all of us that is just meant to play and not worry so much about what is supposed to happen and how things are supposed to be, and be free from the need to over-understand everything. We should have freedom from the idealization, perfectionism and intellectualization of our culture. I think back to the little girl in the photo and I recall that I didn't trust her. I did not trust the embodied version of me, so desiring of a true engagement in life. It's as if I did not believe that was what was actually a valuable way of being. But now I do and I touch base with her all the time. So when you said "inner guidance" in the beginning, I was thinking my guide for this work is that six-year-old version of me that was wanting so badly to be living in and from her body exactly as it was.

I was teaching at the university and a student was in my class who taught yoga and she said to me, "What you're teaching is aligned with yoga philosophy," and she said, "You should come to a yoga class. You would love it."

And I said, "Well, I'm not flexible. I'm the person they put in the back of the dance class—literally, that has happened to me." She responded, "Just come," and it was her yoga class in which I experienced that first feeling of embodiment.

And we studied and then co-created this yoga-based prevention program for ten years and then the doctoral students just came. They wanted to be on the team because at that time no one else was researching yoga as a protective practice.

So, on my team, we all have the desire to share what it means to become more integrated and embodied, because we've experienced the relief in suffering that comes with embodiment and we want to share that experience or pathway with other people.

What's really interesting is the people who are drawn to my lab. My research team are really similar to myself in the way that they're highly driven by the intellectualization of experience and yet passionate about embodiment. Many come into this work present with that same split between their intellectual self and their embodied self. Like me, the spiritual and the material needs are artificially separated. Many of the aspiring researchers I work with have either not experienced the attunement of the material and spiritual self or via trauma or other experiences they were ripped apart from each other.

Critically, we want to figure out in the lab what is happening, how it happened, and what the implications are for prevention and protection of mental health. In this way, we get really intellectual about it.

I mean, it's interesting, I guess. But to have an integrated life and then consider that? That's the stuff. And that's what it is like on the team; when stuff like that happens, we're like, "It's this," and we're like, "Yes!"

It's very joyful. I remember this feeling from marching band. I was in marching band in high school and played trumpet, and when we are all moving together in attunement in a forward march and playing the same beautiful song, just this sense of warmth and feeling of burning pride and love, a fire in your belly and your chest. It's that feeling. It's a very similar feeling when we're coming together with ideas and creating interventions and analyzing data on the research team.

It's an attunement, an integration and a shared physical experience of creation.

I have a dual intellectual process. One of them is the traditional scientific method that I do at work, and I also continue to practice and teach yoga, typically at a studio. I teach four classes a week and I also run a not-for-profit that teaches yoga in the community and we create access to yoga, all separate from my academic work.

I work through various texts (the intellectual approach). I'll go through the whole book and it's kind of like a reading club, but we start the class and I'll read. Often the students will buy the book too and then I'll have them embody the passage, the whole class (the embodied approach). I practice that way, too. I read a lot of Pema Chödrön; I love her work. And so I've worked through quite a few of her books and I've done that many times. I date my notes in the books and often write a few notes—so the books are a bit like a practice journal for me. It's really separate from my research, although it's really not, because, of course, it helps me think of ideas for research.

It really helps me think of ideas that haven't been considered by other researchers because I'm really digging into the yoga philosophy and mindfulness philosophy. All my work, practices and personal study, all help create a more connected, deep and insightful approach to the research.

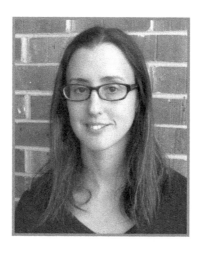

• • ● • •

Marlysa Sullivan is a physiotherapist and yoga therapist with over 15 years of experience working with people suffering with chronic pain conditions. She is Assistant Professor in Yoga Therapy and Integrative Health Sciences at Maryland University of Integrative Health and holds an adjunct position at Emory University, where she teaches the integration of yoga and mindfulness into physical therapy practice in the DPT (Doctor of Physical Therapy) program. She is the author of *Understanding Yoga Therapy: Applied Philosophy and Science for Well-being* and co-editor of *Yoga and Science in Pain Care: Treating the Person in Pain*, as well as several peer-reviewed articles.

Marlysa has supported the professionalization of the field of yoga therapy through the educational standards committee of the International Association of Yoga Therapists (IAYT), further defining the competencies for the field. Marlysa characterizes the yoga therapy workforce development through research and writing. Her current focus is on defining the framework and explanatory model for yoga therapy, based on philosophical foundations and neurophysiological perspectives.

Marlysa Sullivan

I think we must continue to explore the potency of yoga therapy through a deeper lens, really coming underneath to see the thread that brings it altogether. I am sensing into some of the important questions for us to look at, perhaps asking, "What does it mean for these practices to inspire and help create systemic change?"

I was always looking for a much more expansive way of exploring beliefs and spirituality and healing, and how I could practically apply that with people.

As I worked with patients as a physical therapist, I would bring in a little bit of yoga therapy, connecting to one's inner source, one's truth and authenticity, connecting to one's belief. The power of these practices became apparent. So I would say both in my personal healing journey and when I worked with patients, it validated that what I sought to do, what I believed in and what I was being drawn towards was a valid thing.

When I began to work with patients, I was adding to the current. One of the things that really has been clear to me as I worked on my own personal healing, as I worked with students, is that I had that opportunity to start teaching more. So I had all this information, multiple intelligences coming together from my own personal path, from collegial talks with my mentors and friends and from students as I worked in different settings. I was able to see how this work had meaning in many different kinds of settings and many different places.

So it's deepened with my study of Polyvagal theory, eudaimonia and purpose and meaning. I enjoy being able to take all of these different kinds of learnings and cognitive knowledge and ask, "What is the main intention? What is the main purpose? What is the main meaning?"

What do they have to offer? What do Aristotle's teachings have to do with neuroscience and physiology and with Viktor Frankl's teachings and the Bhagavad Gita? The gift of all these languages is that it makes it more accessible to people, so that I can talk to doctors in the language of Aristotle, which they seem to like, or I can talk to people in the language of neuroscience or to people in the language of more spiritual traditions. Because I can see the common thread underneath and speak to that common thread, then the more divergent voices can feel heard and understood and seen.

So I think what I have to offer that river that's moving or that ocean that's moving is the tying together of different voices in a very applicable way. So that's where I see what it is, the way that my life force is putting the intelligence together, the way it flows through me, what it has to offer that current.

When you work with people, you realize that no lineage is going to work for every person. There's no one practice that's going to work for every person, no one breath technique, no one protocol.

It's about being able to come outside what works or doesn't work for you to really see what's underlying. I think for us to build this community and this field, we must ask, "How do we mesh these underlying and aligning findings with these yoga philosophies that are just so amazing and filled with such wisdom? How do we mesh all that with the current ideas that are emerging?"

In order to nurture, as we begin to nurture what it is that our gifts are discovering, our next steps; what is it that I have to offer the world? It's important to do it with a sense of safety.

What has really surprised me and been really powerful to me is just the amazement and wonderment of what life brings to us. That when we're really receptive to it and we allow that too, we allow ourselves to meet it openly and compassionately, things we never thought about, actually arise. Things that we never thought, they emerge. That ability, I feel like that pull that exists in a lot of society is that you have to fit into a box, or you have to always be this one thing. I love the freedom that comes from noticing that contraction and welcoming its opposite and welcoming the ability to just wonder what the next step is. Like I wonder what is going to emerge from this.

I think I've been really surprised in life. I often have thought that when I was a small person, I never could have planned for everything to happen. I couldn't have sat down with a schedule book and said, "On this date, I'll meet this person. On this date, I'll meet this person." Being open to that curiosity and exploration, and by doing what excites you and brings you joy, being open to what needs to come, it will come. So that quality of patience and curiosity, I don't always love the word "faith," but it is kind of a faith. That when you're open and receptive to the world, what emerges is going to be beyond your thinking. It's beyond what your thinking mind can plan.

There's a quote from Viktor Frankl, something like, "What if the question of the meaning of life was reversed?" So instead of me saying, "What is the meaning of this supposed to be?" Instead, maybe life is asking me. So if I'm able to meet life in every moment, life will offer me what my purpose is. To really rest into that power, I think, is really amazing.

Because certainly, I remember someone one time said—it was Doug Keller, he talked about yoga always evolving, it's always been an evolving thing. So yoga has the capacity to absorb and evolve with all the things that we're finding. So finding these neurophysiological principles that align with what yoga has said, it doesn't replace it. It doesn't mean it's exactly the same thing; it's just really cool to see how neurophysiology aligns with it, how Aristotle aligns with it, how we can use all this in different settings with different people. The more we cut that away by saying, "This person's perspective is better, this person's way of teaching is better," we really lose heart. You lose its power and its potency.

So I think to continue to explore its potency through really coming underneath to see the thread that brings it altogether. I think some of the important questions for us to look at, to ask before, but I think what you asked is "What does it mean for these practices to create systemic change?" I know there's a concept and I haven't read that much about it; it's called autonomic synchrony. When I attune my nervous system to a certain way, that has an effect on people around me. So in group settings, we can begin, as we attune and align ourselves in a different frequency, and I don't mean that in some kind of esoteric way, I just mean your autonomic nervous system. As you begin to attune that into a different setting, it's going to effect change larger than yourself. So we can use these ideas in neuroscience, like mirror neurons and autonomic nervous system activations, to begin to give our cognitive minds something to lean on to be able to express these teachings in powerful ways.

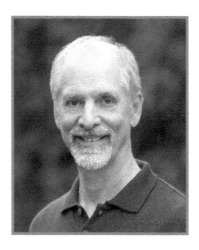

• • • • •

Gary Kraftsow began his study of yoga in India with T.K.V. Desikachar in 1974 and received a Viniyoga Special Diploma from Viniyoga International in Paris, France, in 1988.

Gary opened Maui School of Yoga Therapy in the early 1980s. In 1999, he founded the American Viniyoga Institute™, where he is Director and Senior Teacher.

Gary has successfully developed protocols for two National Institutes of Health studies—"Evaluating Yoga for Chronic Low Back Pain" and "Yoga Therapy for Generalized Anxiety"—as well for the "Mind–Body Stress Reduction in the Workplace" clinical trial for Aetna Insurance Company.

He is the author of two books published by Penguin—*Yoga for Wellness* and *Yoga for Transformation*—and author of four educational DVDs: *Viniyoga Therapy for Low Back, Sacrum and Hips* and *Viniyoga Therapy for Upper Back, Neck and Shoulders*, *Viniyoga Therapy for Depression* and *Viniyoga Therapy for Anxiety*.

Gary Kraftsow

So then I ask, "How do you use breath and introduce the power of sound and chanting and mantra in any language to influence the mind, to influence the emotions and the mind and then to create a relationship with something beyond the mind?"

When I was in my twenties, I was going to go up to the mountain. Desikachar informed me that his father said to tell me that the path of going to the mountain was not relevant. You must go into the world and share this. Do something useful for all beings.

My prayer was: "Help me stay on the path. Help me stay and find a way to manifest it in the world."

Working with the multidimensionality of the human system and the ancient evolved tools helps us create a conscious relationship with ourselves at a multidimensional level. We refine that relationship, so we eliminate sources of suffering at a multidimensional level, while also actualizing our highest potential. All is revealed and transmitted through the ancient traditions.

I think the journey of this work is helping individuals uncover their own truths, the treasure that exists in their heart. In China, the treasure was buried in the hearths and so for me that's a metaphor of the heart and it's already in us. Our job is not to import it from India or China, but to awaken to that treasure already buried inside of us. This is a guiding principle for me in my work with people. We're not converting people, except in helping them wake up to the treasure already within them.

As we come into stillness and continue to do the work of emptying ourselves of ourselves so that we can be in full presence, then creation keeps coming. The new keeps coming.

My life will bring me into contact with world teachers from different traditions. That's just what it's been.

From early on, one of the things that I articulated to myself early in the 1970s was that this is a path in which there is no doubt. As a mature person now, I would say that I had somehow this implicit faith in the truth of these teachings, and when I say these teachings, it's not limited to the yoga training that I was receiving. It was the world's collective understanding that was transmitted through my exposure to world religious traditions. So I became a student of world religion. And my job was to make these teachings alive and real in my own life, and I think that when I was a young man, the first challenge was how do I make a living in society and stay in dharma, stay in integrity with what my inner sort of orientation was to ask how not to compromise. And my teacher said, "Just teach." And it was interesting because when I first started teaching yoga, people came to me with back problems and then they were coming to me with sleep issues and then they were coming to me with depression.

So it naturally evolved; the depth of the work evolved naturally and then, at a certain point, my own unresolved conditions and patterns emerged. I was wanting to be with a woman, and there was this whole community. I lived in Maui back in the seventies. And there was this whole community of people who got into yoga, but what they were into was very different than what I had learned. They were into ashtanga yoga, their guru was a student of my teacher. The tantric movement emerging in Maui was like California sex therapy, yet I had studied Madras tantra. I was afraid of it. I mean, I'm sure I needed it, but it wasn't a tantra that I had learned. So then I took refuge. In that same year, 1976, a Tibetan Lama was sent to establish a dharma center for all sects, to create a new life. So I took refuge with this Lama and served on the Board of Directors of his dharma center for 20 years.

It started in the field of yoga, rooted in personal practice. And that is in the Sadhna. The actual working with ourselves in relationship to ourselves and recognizing that we as human beings are multidimensional and that the Sadhna is multidimensional and what we're doing with yoga Sadhna and yoga practice is creating a conscious relationship with ourselves on a multidimensional level. And then recognizing an expanded understanding of what self is. So I have a conscious, whole feel for asana as a means of helping us create a conscious relationship with our functional anatomy so that we can create stability and strength and range of motion, and maintain it through life. But we're not just that; we're also an autonomic nervous system. So the field of pranayama is like creating a conscious relationship with our autonomic nervous system so that we can create sympathetic, parasympathetic regulation and it goes on like that.

And our relationship with our changing emotions, our relationship with our stories, the stories we tell ourselves about ourselves, our narrative that should really predict today what's going on in our world and our interpretations. And then our relationship to each other—sort of the expanded notion of self. And so I feel like for me it's been a process of using Sadhna to understand and then to work to refine my relationship to my self, which is an expanded self through Sadhna practice. And from there, then I start communicating back to people. I think of two sorts of protocols that inspire people to do something at a new level. One is pain and suffering and another is a mysterious, deep inner longing or interest or passion for truth. And so a lot of the people I work with are suffering and they want to find a way of refining, of relieving their suffering. In our path, it's finding a way of understanding yourself, finding out what you're doing habitually that's either causing or complicating the healing, causing the suffering or maintaining it.

We ask, "What can you do to stop doing those things and what can you start doing that can help you find a healing or transformation?" And so I think that if I understood your question correctly, for me it was the landing point and then bringing; it is through communicating with people that are looking for either relief from pain or connecting to something beyond themselves.

So it's our thoughts, our mind, our self-concept and the narrative that we're telling ourselves about ourselves and the world around us. It's our changing feelings and emotions, moods, but mostly that feeling quality. And then it's our behavior, our actions which are related to our wills and all of that kind of comes from our desires which themselves come from our conditioning.

My prayer was help me stay on the path. Help me stay and find a way to manifest it in the world.

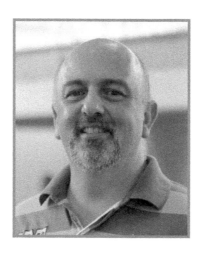

• • ● • •

Danilo Forghieri Santaella is one of the first researchers in yoga physiology in Brazil, working with yoga teaching and research at the University of São Paulo. He teaches practical and theoretical classes for the elderly and the university community, as well as applying his acquired knowledge to research and to strengthening yoga's respectability among the scientific and medical community. He teaches Applied Physiology in postgraduate Yoga and Yoga Therapy courses. His main research field is the interaction between mind and body, with special emphasis on the influences of yoga on psychobiological variables/markers. Investigations have addressed the following interventions and variables: the aging process, yoga as therapy, relaxation, breathing exercises (pranayama), physical exercise, hypertension, post-exercise blood pressure, heart-rate variability, EEG, evoked potentials, aging brain, functional connectivity, stress, sleep quality and quality of life. Danilo is also connected to Kaivalyadhama Yoga Institute (India), and represented South America in the first World Consortium for Yoga Therapy in Japan (2018).

Danilo Forghieri Santaella

Through my papers and my investigations, I try to point out the biggest inner changes, the biggest biological changes that yoga may offer. You will have them only if you practice yoga in a very subtle way, in a very easygoing way. Exercise: the more you practice, the more you get tired. Asana: the more you practice, the more you rest.

We tend to speak about how things are due to changes and that we should adapt. And in yoga, we always say, don't get so attached to stuff, everything is transitory, like in Buddhism. But I believe that sometimes we don't actually live it in the true sense. And this period that we are passing through now is forcing us to adapt. It's forcing us to let go; it's forcing us to develop a different way of reaching people because we, as therapists or as yoga teachers, we need to get in touch with people. That's how we practice our profession; we exert our profession through the contact with people. But now the contact with the people is like this video call—what we're doing now in "corona time."

One thing I really like to pay attention to and getting in touch with is to pay attention to the breath flow, which breaks boundaries of the inner space with the outer space.

It actually makes us, and are we getting the idea that there's no inside and there's no outside. There's no difference between me, you or somebody, or anybody who may be around. It doesn't matter if he's black or white or fat or strong or thin or old or young or an engineer or a yoga teacher or a prisoner—air goes inside everybody. Air doesn't choose hearts, air doesn't choose intentions, air doesn't choose formations, air doesn't choose if you're gay, if you're hetero or anybody, anything else.

There's no difference between people; there's no difference between beings. We're all here, we all share the same air, the same earth, and we may have the same elements, we may have a mission, or we may not. But if we shared an idea of getting together, we have to respect differences and qualities and finish with expectations, and this leads normally to a reciprocity and relationship. And if we have none, even the yoga practice gets better. Even short contact gets a better flow and we find some harmony.

My inspiration came from my mother. She was a very, very interesting woman—she's passed on, passed away now, since 2005. And she went early—she was 60, very young. She used to read a lot about psychology; she used to talk a lot with her friends, in her home. I used to pay attention; I liked to listen to them speaking and talking about life and existential subjects. When I got to the university, in a physical education bachelor's degree program here in Brazil, I was in a group that got together in the houses of the other group members to meditate.

This group was formed by some friends of my mother's. They believed that you can build a better future by spreading good, by spreading good energy—what you think, yet mostly your behavior. Meditations that would put you in contact with higher beings in the universe. I did get something really interesting from that and it pointed me in the direction of yoga. They believed that, and they still do—the group's still going on, yet I'm not a part of this anymore. We actually had some yoga practices in the community. But for real, what really happened is a discovery that this side of my mind, which is prone to trying and getting actions to do better, to do well with people, through action, also lives along with another very rational side in my brain, which doesn't accept anything explained or not explained. I have a very inner-oriented nature of investigation where I go to the deeper stuff.

I got my internship in meditation and my other friend went to be an intern in the yoga class in the sports center of the same university, University of São Paulo, where I work now. And we were studying different stuff and she knew about this side I have in meditation, and she said, "You should go and try a yoga class." And I said, "No, but I'm stiff, I can't put my feet behind my ears." When I went, the first class, the teacher, Marcos, my yoga master, he said, "Okay, now try to stretch comfortably."

And he gave many references of research during his class and I said, "I'm liking it even more now."

And then I just couldn't stop practicing; it saved me during my master's from having a heart attack, I'm really sure about it.

And then I was so convinced about this good that yoga can do to people. And when I looked around, even my mother, who gave me all the inspiration to go for it. When I went to the yoga class, she said, "There you go, to make your 'OM' again."

Making jokes, I said, "Even like you, mom." And ultimately, she became a student in one of my classes. It was really nice. My worst student, but she was there.

That inquisitive nature I have has led me not only to a biochemistry internship, but also to an exercise physiology internship. And when I finished my undergrad, I definitely wanted to continue studying. But not only studying because I wanted to know more, but because it was something of an ego quest. I wanted to help yoga become more respected in society. It was 1996. Imagine when I started, I studied for my master's degree in the School of Medicine here at the University of São Paulo. One of the most conservative schools, old-fashioned schools that we have here. And I'm from physical education, so of course medical people don't look up to us.

And if we are open to it, use what your heart says and the potential to be anything we want in life. If I'm really, really determined now that I can do something, I will.

I wanted to understand the functioning of the body. But I didn't actually; it's a kind of childish way of choosing because I didn't want to kill animals during my studies.

If I had gone to medical school, I would have killed pigs, I would have killed dogs during surgery, practicing, and it would be really sad for me.

Why not go into physical therapy, then? Those days, in the beginning, I didn't want to work with suffering; I preferred the positive side of health. So I went to physical education. But as I have gone deeper in my studies, I started researching how to make ill people better. And then it took me to therapy.

My yoga teacher started to do social work for the House Foundation, which is for kids, male and female, under 21. After that, they go to prison or they go to the streets. And he started teaching yoga inside there, that institution. And I was one of the volunteers, along with many others, and this work still goes on.

And I didn't feel so comfortable because I wanted to believe that what I was doing would change their lives, but I couldn't really believe it. I was not such a believer in the capacity that those boys would have to become good if they were really bad. I should have the opportunity to try to not do the bad stuff that they did and try to change and everything—that's what we believe in, as yoga researchers, yeah? But back then, I said, "If I'm not so good at doing this, I prefer to try to do better for people in the biological health side of health, not in this sociological one."

And then my academic tutor said, "But you can't write yoga in your project; you're going into therapy and we are going into medicine!"

I said, "Oh, cool, but can I research yoga and not say it is yoga?"

She said, "OK, yeah, let's try and find a way to do the research."

So that was the beginning, and the research was to be in hypertension. So if I could find something in yoga that would help treat hypertension, she would guide me through it. Savasana was the obvious choice. I put together a project that was approved, yet I couldn't put in the word "savasana," nor could I put the word "yoga" in it either.

We called it "relaxation." Two and a half years later, I published our findings in the *Journal of the American College of Sports Medicine.* My research became well represented all over the world. I went on to my PhD and then, as you said, if you follow your path, truly believing that you're doing it in your dharmic way, stuff will happen. Interestingly, many other people started doing similar investigations at the same time.

But now, if you go to PubMed and you put a search for yoga with no date limit, you will have 6000 or so papers. But if you ask for only the last five years, you'll have at least half of it. It's like an exponential curve. So, in my PhD project, I was able to say that we are going to study pranayama and yoga in elderly people! We published in *British Medical Journal,* the open version. It was the first year of the journal, back in 2010, and in the second and third year, we saw a significant impact factor.

If we don't listen to our inner voice and we try to build a way to our self-development, yet it's not our dharmic path, we're not listening.

This may all be connected to all these influences, and sometimes when you just pay attention to things that are happening around you, you get those clues, you get those signs and stuff starts to happen, like all of a sudden. I never had dreamed about the possibility of going to India. And then when I decided I would make a plan to go to India in five years, in five months I was there.

The universe just has to rearrange it for it to happen because it had to happen.

So I think that I will be more true to myself while trying to build a very nice body of knowledge for people to beat stress or to beat hypertension or to beat traumatic stress, depression or something like that.

So, if you get the second sutra eventually, people like to believe it's the first one, but it's actually the second that matters. Well, the first one really helps too. Hatha yoga means yoga is a self-discipline and it's now. So, if you're not willing to change, don't start. But if you start, it's for easing the mind, it's for healthiness, for getting into a place in which our ego goes back and serves us, not as individuals, but as a "*we.*" Coming from "*me*" to "*we,*" as you so fantastically point out. And this will give way to our will. Sometimes my English just doesn't let me speak what I want to...

Our egos will surrender to the highest wills if we are gentle to ourselves. If we get to that oceanic sensation during the asanas. So, my quest comes together, my investigative nature meets my practical yoga practice.

You shouldn't practice more than 45 or 50 minutes of asanas, because if you do, you get lazy. And asanas are meant to prepare you for pranayama, which is meant to prepare you for meditation. And if you practice asana as asana, it is already a kind of meditation. And see my second latest paper, it was a really nice one in *Frontiers in Aging Neuroscience.* We proved that people who practice yoga in a traditional way and they are over 60 years old, get the connectivity of the frontal part of the brain. They practice yoga for at least eight years, at least twice a week, it's not so much practice, one hour per day, per practice, and they get the connectivity of the frontal part of the brain, with the back part of the brain increased and preserved.

The importance is the link between the back part of the brain and the front part of the brain. As we age, normally our brain shrinks. You just can't deny it, but you can make it happen slower. The cortex is where all the main connections of the brain happen, and it is responsible for formatting our consciousness. And if this part of the brain talks to this part, which talks to this part, we call it brain connectivity. And there are different networks that come into play in different tasks that we're doing. One of them is called the default mode network. The default mode network is a part of the brain that is formed by many parts and that's the one I investigated. It becomes very active when we are resting.

Yoga has to be practiced in a traditional way, asana as asana, not as exercise, because we found our results in people who were matched to a control group, which had the same amount of physical exercise as the yoga group. The difference reported in our findings is all about the self-attention, the awareness component of yoga.

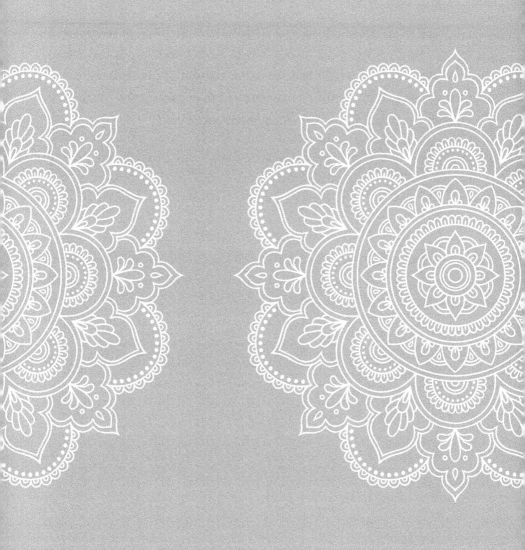

VI

Reflections on
Participatory Action

*Returning to rediscover the deeper
shared roots, naming the magic
of the ancient forms of true
connection, staying simple.*

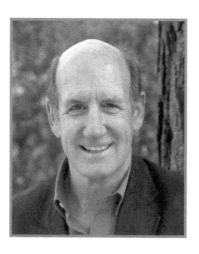

•••••

Richard C. Miller is a clinical psychologist, author, researcher, yogic scholar and spiritual teacher who has devoted his life to integrating Western psychology and neuroscience with the ancient non-dual wisdom teachings of yoga, Tantra, Advaita, Taoism and Buddhism. He is the founder and president of iRest Institute, co-founder of the International Association of Yoga Therapists, and a founding member and past president of the Institute for Spirituality and Psychology.

Publications include *iRest Meditation: Restorative Practices for Health, Healing and Well-Being*, *The iRest Program for Healing PTSD* and *Yoga Nidra: The Meditative Heart of Yoga*. Richard serves as a research consultant for iRest Yoga Nidra Meditation, studying its efficacy on issues such as sleep, PTSD, pain and chemical dependency within diverse populations. He continues the inquiry with research on iRest's efficacy for enhancing resiliency and wellbeing. The U.S. Army Surgeon General and the Defense Centers of Excellence have recognized iRest as a complementary program for healing chronic pain and PTSD.

Richard C. Miller

I think the underlying driving force here behind all of us, we're all searching for love, to feel deeply seen, connected, a sense of being heard and a sense of belonging. It's not just a belonging inside, but with life itself, and then with the greater culture around us, so we don't feel isolated. Even though we may be like we're doing now in this time of COVID, in social isolation or distancing, we keep that sense of connectedness. To me, the life that I'm living, the mission I've been sent on, that I feel deeply involved in, is really that work to help people first connect to themselves, then connect to the people around them and understand what their mission is.

Whenever we forget our underlying wholeness, or when we begin to separate from ourself in some way, we don't attend to a particular emotion that's arising or a particular thought. When we separate in any way within ourselves from wholeness or ourself, it will always give rise to anxiety, fear and the feeling that something is amiss.

We are all deeply, deeply interconnected. We need to keep taking moments of our day, as I do, to feel that sense of interconnectedness. Especially during challenging times, which can make us feel sometimes isolated or alone; in fact, we are never alone. We are first always with another, ourself, and we can feel that deep interconnectedness, both with those people far and near, but also with the trees, the earth, the plants, and know that there is a sense of harmony here.

Nature was always a part of my life. I didn't think anything of it. It was just there. Then later on, when I was 13, I happened to be on a vacation visiting my grandma. It was an evening, and I was taking a walk. I lay down, and I looked up into the evening sky, and as a teenager might do, and I did, I wondered, "I wonder where the end of the universe is."

Later, at the end of a yoga class, what I now know is that the teacher taught a rudimentary yoga nidra meditation practice. Again, I had that same experience that I had at 13. I walked out, I felt myself as the trees, the stars. I didn't feel any sense of separation.

A depression, an isolation that I had been carrying with me from my teenage years, completely vanished. I felt that innate sense of connectedness, both with myself, but also all this—my place in the universe. That spurred what I call now a great vow to rise up in me spontaneously: what has been happening in these different experiences? What are practices that I can engage, and how do I learn more? With that intention—I think intentions are so strong when they come from that deep place of spontaneity—it drew me to different teachers, who slowly helped me experience different practices, and begin to fall into these moments of unitedness on a regular basis.

Looking back, that's now how I understand it. What I felt in the moment was a sense of "I don't know how to do this social thing." I started to feel more and more isolated within myself, even though I had good friends, and enjoyed experiences growing up. It cultivated with me a deep sense of separateness. That question of "What's going on, and how can I find my way?" kept coming up in different ways. I had those different experiences with the trees, or looking up into the universe, or later on with my first teacher. We were sitting together, and she really helped lead me, through her own presence, back into my own presence. I would then recapture that sense of unity.

It kept sparking within me that this was available and that I could find a way back, I would say, to the sense of wholeness. At first, though, like I think probably with everyone, I was looking outside for it. I feel gifted in that all my teachers kept turning me back in.

I began to look at what are the underlying threads that all these spiritual traditions hold in common. I started dipping into Sufism. I was studying the work of Gurdjieff. I was still involved in Christianity. I started looking at the Judaism roots. Buddhism, I sat in Zen, Mahayana, and then continued my yoga.

I kept coming back to this image of a well. I realized I was digging lots of wells, and I might never reach water. That pondering helped me realize: "Let me come back and dig one well. Let's do the yoga well."

I really started anchoring into yoga, still pulling in my Buddhist roots and Christian roots, but exploring the teachings experientially. I'm thankful for my teachers. They weren't trying to make me become an intellect. They were saying, "What is your actual moment-to-moment experience? What's happening inside of you?" They kept turning me back into myself.

What I see now is that underlying essence, that life force, it was always guiding me. My job was to attune and listen more and more deeply. I loved a quote—I think it was one of the Presidents; it might have been FDR or Coolidge: "Comparison is the thief of joy. Comparison is the thief of joy." All of my teachers kept coming back and saying, "Don't compare. Stop looking out, keep going in. That guiding force is what you want to align with."

That brought me then to that moment, I would say in 1995, or whenever it was, when that light switch came on. All the teachings I would say came together in that moment, and I really felt that underlying quality of, call it essence, wholeness, non-duality, whatever you want to call it. It just landed in a very simple way that said, "The search is done. Now it's really about living it." I moved, I would say in that moment, from being a seeker to a finder, and then my job really became "What's the expression that this force wants to live through me?"

That's when I was approached back in 2004 by the military, who said, "Change the name, because we don't know what to do with this name, yoga and meditation. We're soldiers, we do mission. We don't do yoga." That's when I came up with the name Integrative Restoration—iRest. What I've come to realize, these practices really do help us become a fully potentialized human being. That we're unique in our expressions as a human being, but we need to become very integrated in our ability to work with our emotions, our thoughts, our body. We have a body and a mind.

Go to the source of where you feel the separation is arising within yourself. Use the emotions and the thoughts and the body's sensations as pointers back to their source, which is going to reveal to you where you're separating. Heal that sense of separation, and you'll find what you're looking for.

Nature would be thanking us for finally getting the message that she's been sending to us for decades now, to come back into that sense of connectedness and harmony.

I'm a pragmatic optimist. My optimist knows that we'll eventually get it all right. My pragmatic nature: it's going to take probably a very long time. I'm in for the long haul.

My life mission, I would say, is to help people discover not just their connectedness back with themselves, but that interconnectedness with everyone around them.

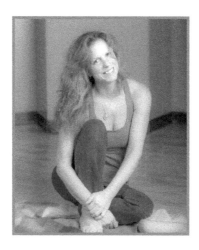

• • ● • •

Helene Couvrette is a certified yoga therapist with IAYT (International Association of Yoga Therapists). With over 22 years' experience, Helene specializes and is certified in pain care yoga and trauma-informed yoga therapy, and yoga education.

She founded H~OM Yoga Center/School in 2007, where she teaches group classes, offers private one-on-one yoga therapy sessions and is the lead educator in her 200-hour, 300-hour and 800-hour Yoga Therapy Program.

Helene is the president of MISTY—Montreal International Symposium on Therapeutic Yoga—which she co-founded in 2011. Helene is also a proud and dedicated mom of four amazing kids, grandma to one sweet little girl and another grandchild on the way!

Helene Couvrette

I love the first sutra of Pantajali, "now the practice of yoga."

I was just talking with a friend today who is having a very hard time with the impact of COVID. She's stuck in New Mexico but lives in Vermont and it just hit her. She's been enjoying her vacation and extended it, saying, "Oh, I'll just stay here." Yes, but now the practice of yoga. I think I wake up every morning and every other sutra following are the other steps. But first we just have to land and say just that. In everything I do, in every way I behave, in the way I listen, in the way I talk, in the way I walk, I strive. I don't manage it all the time, but I strive to just leave it to just the basics. We just have to practice it.

I wanted to do more yoga. I don't have the self-discipline to do it alone as much as I want to, but to share. I have four children, so the sharing was something that I really wanted to do so I could do more. I was wanting more by giving more, and at the time I knew a woman who had breast cancer and I asked a few of my friends, "Do you guys want to help me practice teaching? I could teach you guys some yoga," and the friend with the cancer said, "We could do it in my basement." I started teaching yoga to four people in a basement with a woman who had cancer who did die a few years after that.

Yes, that was the beginning.

I used to teach out of a community center before I opened my center, and on the registration, I asked a question: "What brings you to yoga? What are you looking for?"

I had stretching, get stronger, get more balance, get fit, a few things, but for everyone, it might have been the only thing, it was always get fit and relax. Get stronger and release stress. That releasing of stress seemed to be always on there.

My teaching, I guess by listening and hearing these stories, it was like whatever we're doing physically doesn't matter. It's not the poses, and I often ask at the beginning of my class, "What are you here for? What got you up and got you here?" At the end of the class, "Did you get it? Did it have anything to do with Warrior 1? Did it have anything to do with this sequence or this particular pose or the other?"

Then when someone had brain cancer and came to classes and she passed away, I thought, "Why did I charge her money?" I started to say, "If anyone has cancer and is in treatment, you don't have to pay."

To me there's no beginning and end between my suffering and what I get out of it and their suffering and what they get out of it.

Life has a fabulous way of happening. I'm thinking at this time again, it's a chance, it's a gift really. I think that because seeing people suffer, because I suffered, many different things happened in my life that yoga was there to help me ground, and I saw it ground others as I shared it and then I grounded more in sharing it.

I was a connecting force of the people. I was a face of it. My partner at the time was doing websites but I was making this interaction.

I started teacher training and I heard myself teaching the meaning, the purpose behind all these shapes we happen to want to teach because teachers come in at the 200 level. I now do the 300 and I started to hear myself now do more of the teaching, so my teaching grows within me. I'm not just teaching the class. Now I'm teaching trainees. Now I'm teaching them all the other stuff that is not really in the details in a regular yoga class. All the philosophies, I always start with that. I say, "There's no point. We'll do some postures, but until you really understand the philosophy, then you can really use the postures to do more with."

If you think of yoga, you can teach the poses and even teach the philosophy, but I like teaching with stories of how it applies in my life.

I don't mind baring my soul and my struggles. That's yoga to me, that we're reaching a person through all the layers.

Not just teaching them about the layers but teaching them to their layers.

By connecting with others and seeing what they're doing, by watching the shift in me and in world. My intention behind the MISTY [Montreal International Symposium of Therapeutic Yoga] conference is to leave my mark on this world. How can I leave an imprint that will make a difference?

I think that human society can thrive if we can keep taking the walls down between the differences of medicine and yoga, which has happened over the last ten years. It's been incredible over the last 20 years to see it. As I evolved, I've watched it evolve as well.

I feel that everybody who comes in my path, everybody I choose for MISTY, I call them, I want a conversation via FaceTime, I want to feel their energy. It matters because it's an energy between the weekend of these dozen presenters and myself. Together we're creating the energy of what MISTY is. I put out the platform. We have a Friday faculty dinner. We have a lot of fun. We go outside. There's no separateness. There's no dualism. We're all there creating that energy.

Then to hear people being so grateful and to feel this mission of trying to help people, for me it's a simple mission. I want to help people who suffer. The way I feel is we have to educate. Yoga people, medical people, and then bring them together. Take the divide down and unite. In that way, we can help people who suffer because it all goes back to that person in the basement. And everybody else who shared their stories.

It's just the impact of that "something"...you're just swimming along and then all of a sudden, oh, that's happening because of this conference. This is happening. The things that can happen because it was not something that was in my first intention. I just wanted to get the medical and yoga world together, but I'm finding that that's happening but so are other things happening.

How we can all create something; that drives me to keep creating. I just feel this tradition is uniting. It is about uniting within ourselves, our own mind, body, spirit, and everybody together uniting. And seeing what can happen.

I love the idea of being surprised. I love the idea of being in awe. I love the idea of not knowing. I say often to my children, "You have no idea what can happen anytime, anywhere, to anyone." It could be tragic, like COVID. But it can also be amazing. It's like I can't wait to see what happens next time.

I try to go with an openness. People often will, when I ask them to present, "What's your theme?" And they go, "I don't know." I ask them to send me four choices of subjects. Everybody does two. I love puzzles, so I'll lay it all out on a sheet and I'll mix and match—those ones will work, and there it is. Just to let it happen more organically, and then just letting life surprise me.

What comes to mind right now is John Lennon's song "Imagine." I think that when my stillborn, when I lost that baby, I remember saying, "This is not the end of my story," so I got pregnant for the fifth time and had my fourth child, Tessa, which means fourth. I say that in the tragedy of losing this stillborn boy, I grieved it, but that ability to just imagine that it's a domino effect. Because of this, everything else fell into place.

I think that for the readers out there, I would say this. In your darkest time, imagine that you will look back and that the dominoes set up because of this dark time will have a purpose. It doesn't mean that only good will come out of it. But that the path is laid out and not every stone can be right. Imagine in your darkest time that this too will pass. Imagine that there will come a step that becomes lighter and brighter. Then darker ones will come. Imagine that you'll be fine. That you'll be fine, and that every life... Something has to happen every day. It can't all be good, but something has to happen.

If we can just know that some days are going to be darker and some days are going to be lighter, but in the dark ones just imagine the lighter one will come. Visualize it, because where your brain is going to go, where your thoughts are going to go, this is what you're going to feel viscerally.

Grieve when you need to grieve. I think what happens sometimes, I would say to the young readers and any reader, is when we get in a dark place, we imagine it'll always be like this. Our imagined sense is "When's it ever going to end?" As opposed to imagining it will end, and what will I do when it does?

I wrote a post on Facebook and said, "This is an opportunity to shift gears, reassess. Once it's over, what will you bring with you? What will you bring with you, through this COVID time, what are you going to bring with you?" I'm walking more. I've been wanting to walk more. I have the time, so I'm walking more. I'm going to bring with me, "I'm going to continue to walk more." Whatever it is for anyone, what will you bring with you? Sometimes those darker places are times to just reassess.

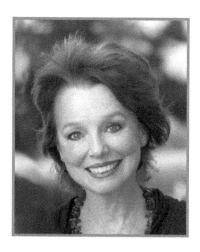

• • ● • •

Camille Maurine is a teacher, meditation mentor, dancer and the author of *Meditation Secrets for Women* and *Meditation 24/7*, written with her husband, Dr. Lorin Roche. In addition to her four-plus decades of dance, yoga and meditation, Camille's integrative approach draws upon training in various healing arts, including the study of Jungian depth psychology and Continuum Movement. She and Lorin have also been cross-pollinating their discoveries and insights and co-creating their approach during their 38 years of relationship. Camille is on the faculty of Esalen Institute, 1440 Multiversity, Kripalu Center for Yoga and Health, SAND Science and Nonduality and The Shift Network. She is the creator of Moving Theater of the Soul, a transformational creative process. Camille often performs excerpts from *The Radiance Sutras*, Lorin Roche's translation of the Vijnana Bhairava Tantra, an ancient meditation text.

Camille Maurine

It's in paying attention that allows it to grow. It just wants to be met. And then it just gushes with wisdom and gushes with insight and gushes with our next organic natural unfolding. So, rather than imposing, it's the listening and welcoming. I do think when we give ourselves the chance, it is as though we start listening to the voice of the soul. There's the individual's expression of that. But there's also the sense that it can be a very tangible step when we learn the art of allowing the energies to flow more freely through us.

My primary metaphor is dance, that everything is a dance. And well, I grew up a very serious little girl. I was always feeling the call and the curiosity about the essence that was behind all of the teachings. When I discovered dance as my first medium, and it was actually exactly at the same time that I was getting initiated into meditation and then yoga, that exploration of dance, modern dance in particular, but studying ethnic forms was where I came out positive. And then experiencing many, many different spiritual traditions.

It's like my dance is my teacher; it's continually teaching me every moment of the day and then meditation is also informing me.

I didn't have any great plan. I was curious and I was following the creative urge and inviting people to come and explore with me. "Let's see what happens, then if you are interested, I can tell you more of the influences that come forward."

I started having a lot of the subtle movement that I was discovering, very subtle movement in meditation, that spontaneous mood. The understanding that what we call a body is actually not limitation. Where we start to go beyond the collective conventional ideas of what it is to be a human being. So the work took me from kind of an airy spiritual refuge to going deep, deep into the soul. Deep into the primordial energies. And one of my inner teachers became the singing dragon about the routes of the unearthing of the deep feminine wisdom that had been buried in the West.

Then, around the tips of two things, two meetings happened almost concurrently. One was with something called Continuum founded by Emilie Conrad. I was immersed in that and having revelations and then even more revelations about subtle movement and our biological resonance with all of life. She became a primary teacher of embodiment, dancing with this movement of energy that we are.

I met Lorin (Roche) almost exactly around the same time. When Lorin and I met, we discovered that we had so much in common in terms of our integrated embrace to everything, embracing the depths of emotion and the questions of "How do I come to meet myself and the wild and wondrous energies that are here?"

That also started sparking that curiosity about love and what it is to be intimate, which for me was a personal journey coming from experiences of isolation. So those are the primary relationships, you could say, that started to interpenetrate, like you say, to co-create, to co-evolve.

For as long as I can remember, I felt deeply. I ended up being sensitized to the body of humanity. There's always been a sense of something evolving. There's been this sense of, as the decades go on, that something is evolving in us particularly right now and we're all playing a part in that. And my sense, as I say in this, is invoking the eldering wisdom years that both Lorin and I are very aware is happening. There's a global interaction and awakening and sharing going on now. It's very much a sense of honoring the new needs arising now.

It's important to honor these needs because individuality is playing its part, it's essential, and we're all needed now. And so that understanding now comes through things like books and workshops and recordings that serve to be a resource, a place that people can go to for discovery, to allow that unfolding evolutionary movement to have its way.

Nature has gone wild, so finding those places in us that have been overly domesticated or really changed is important. How have we been separated from that natural source? And that is general and also archetypal, this feeling of connection and that we're all in this together. Those are the classic feminine wisdom gifts. Honoring the body. You know that many spiritual traditions imply that it's about transcending; that's a very tricky notion because everything that we experience is actually arising sometimes in very subtle clues.

So that sense of coming to meet those places and they will come up, for example, in meditation, the aches from the stories, the regrets, the longings, the desires, all of which ultimately are the touch of love trying to get our attention.

And so the primary skill is to ask, "How can I come to meet those places inside of myself?" with enormous tenderness for the self and for this condition of being human on the one hand—what a mystery that is!

I have a body of work called Akinesthetics with a capital A. Akinesthetics was the revelation that we are all this glorious unfolding tapestry, artwork of the divine, you could say. It's the sacred energies of how to see through fresh eyes and to come to meet oneself with a kind of appreciation, to come to meet in terms of the way to meet one another, to come to meet one another with "Wow, look at who you are."

So how do I come to meet and feel what's underneath the wellspring?

It sort of feels obvious. The need seems so obvious and the opposite is so exaggerated on earth right now and it's so painful, so painful. So we are being called into dependence. Really getting in it. I think now

I'm getting this Shakti shimmer. Whatever nature is doing with this virus, we're having this opportunity to have the sacred pause and then to realize, holy moly, actually we're dependent on each other on the other side of the world. We're in the global connect. Things like this make that global nervous system open up, allowing communication even while we're all sheltering at home.

So that sense of the interdependence, the sense of coming back and into the way that we are a part of nature. We are part of Nature's body. Can we feel into it? So what arises in me in terms of caring for our environment, caring for one another, is that we need one another.

I cannot imagine a day starting without giving myself the freedom to meditate. Even though I'm a dancer, it's usually a sitting practice. I always give myself the freedom to do whatever that can be expressing the energies coming through. A lot of my own journey and a lot of what I incorporate into the practice is expression because that's a way of allowing energies to move with creative attention.

Being able to give my body again to those energies allows them to move into integration. So because then we're filled with the shock, we're filled with apprenticeship where we can feel the actual life force.

When we learn how to pay attention to that, to give attention, to bring attention to that, for me it becomes more of a way of being in the world every day. I feel like I'm being informed in the meditations as something coming to meet my inspiration, but also for anything aching in my heart. And then I make sure that I'm keeping my energies physically moving, whether it's a dance, being in nature, walking around here or various kinds of yoga.

There can be a sense of necessity of remembering, like soul remembering, a kind of sense of "Here I am with this individual with certain longings, certain desires and ways that I love and what I love, very individual." And it can be like a continual remembering, "Oh yes, that is who I am." That is part of who I am. And at the same time, there can be this kind of "You feel like, I think there is a collective movement of individually and together we're feeling like a call because it's so needed."

This was so way before corona. Now we've been building the intensity and we could think of it as a kind of perturbation to inspire a new, simpler, more elegant form.

We don't know how it will go; we don't know where we've come to. But that kind of remembering is part of our inner practices. Embodiment practices helped so much because, again, they make us feel part of this life that I am. There are different breath practices or asana or movement or subtle, spontaneous mudra.

What happens to me all the time is I just see it in my heart. There is where gestures arise, where a kind of subliminally sourced gestures arise. But there is that feeling, like when we're meditating or tuning in to ourselves to this magnificent expression, that I am really allowing that to take form.

And then we become aware of the form and go, "Oh, I see, this means something to me. This means something to me."

So there's a loop. You keep discovering what that is. And then I do think that we feel as if there's a call of the future and that call of our future self, the one that we're becoming, and in a way, it's going to be a big surprise. You can't really predict and engineer exactly, but we can feel that call and pick up and take our next little movement of "What does it mean for me to say yes to that?"

How do I say yes? How do I feel simultaneously because I'm going to just say that it's important to have our sense of our own sovereignty? Meaning that no one really knows what we should do or be, yet we do. But how do I tune into that? That's where all of our practices come in and also our connection together with the global and collective field or smaller groups coming together in smaller groups, coming together with one other and having this inquiry, like we don't know where this conversation is going.

It's like, wow, how fun and let me feel deeply from my heart. Let me speak my heart. I feel what my truth is; let me feel the intrinsic power, meaning my natural pre-existing sense of power and freedom.

I'm shedding the things that feel like they are just too small for me now. They served a purpose and I'm needing to unfold beyond them. We can sense that it's really just right here. So that call of the future, we can feel something's unfolding me. Life itself is right here, is giving us its whispered visions. And sometimes we get a big revelation. "Wow! This is it." Like when I took my first dance class: "Wow! I'm going to shift from theater to dance." So sometimes we get to experience things like that.

I have the opportunity to be in communion and communication with someone that...what they say a lot is that they feel permission to be themselves and the capital E Essence as well. And that the intimacy that I share with another arises from it to continual intimacy with the self. What is that? And that's a practice. How do I be in that loving awareness and that loving touch with myself, no matter what is going on? How I am listening deeply to myself allows me to listen more deeply with you.

And there's this sense of us listening, sensing together. So it may not be that there's a program that I'm sharing. This is the way, but I can say I can support, and I can encourage you and offer some hints and experiences—contexts from that deeper communion.

I don't think of myself as a leader. Other people call me a leader. Because then it's like, "Do this." I don't know. It seems like to me. I am, I suppose, but I don't think of myself that way nor have I ever. I just share beginning contexts and like that exploration.

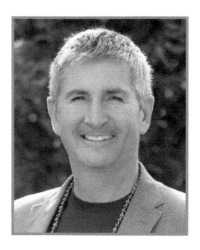

• • ● • •

Neil Pearson is a physical therapist, yoga therapist and Clinical Assistant Professor at the University of British Columbia, teaching in the physiotherapy and pain medicine sub-specialty programs. He is a consultant to the BC Medical Association, to Lifemark's 300+ Canadian rehab clinics, and to Pain BC, Canada's premier nonprofit transforming the way pain is understood and treated.

Neil is founding chair of the Physiotherapy Pain Science Division in Canada, recipient of the Canadian Pain Society's Excellence in Interprofessional Pain Education award, and faculty in four yoga therapist programs. Neil has authored a patient education ebook, *Understand Pain, Live Well Again* (2008); a book chapter "Yoga Therapy" in Thompson and Brooks, *Integrative Pain Management* (2016); numerous journal articles on yoga and pain, including a recent white paper for the International Association of Yoga Therapists, "Yoga Therapy and Pain: How Yoga Therapy Serves in Comprehensive Integrative Pain Management," and "How It Can Do More" (2020); and co-authored/edited the textbook *Yoga and Science in Pain Care: Treating the Person in Pain* (2019).

Neil Pearson

In part, because it's so hard to try to push it out to the world without people thinking that you're saying it wrong. And that's not what I'm trying to say; what I'm trying to say is that we can evolve this, we can take the yoga teaching further around pain. Yoga teaching says this is it. But we're continuing within yoga to treat pain as if it's something that doesn't fit the rules of all the other yoga teachings.

The first initiation would absolutely be the end of the yoga classes that I had started in Vancouver. It was a place called the Wandering Yogi and it was a husband and wife who ran it. There was an opportunity at the end of the class. We would sit down, and we'd have tea and we would talk. What I realized was that this felt like home in a way that the conversation was inquisitive and it was candid. It just was this sharing of these ideas of experiences during the class. We'd just talk about that stuff.

I'd never experienced that openness to be able to just talk about your experience from anything actually in life. Again, it reminded me of, one of the things it really reminded me of was when I was working in the hospitals. I worked in intensive care, both neonatal intensive care but also adult intensive care.

It reminded me a lot of the language of the palliative care workers. So this hospital was in Sudbury, Ontario and the Grey Nuns had been associated with starting the hospital and the state affiliated with it. They essentially were the holders of wisdom and compassion and would take care of people in the worst of possible times, both the staff and the patients there. It reminded me of their language. Their language and their love and their openness, right, and acceptance.

But the other place was really once again the opportunity to speak freely about ideas and just share them in a much more deep way when I was doing the yoga philosophy training.

Once again, when you said it, what it reminded me of, both times it actually felt like this is who I am, this is what I want to do, right, this is where I feel good.

That's not the same kind of feeling that I've had in the academic world or even in the healthcare world. Most of the times there's not an openness.

I think one of the biggest things around healthcare is the need to be right and to know it is so... That's what we're all trying to be and do, right?

I think it really comes down to love. It's love, it's acceptance, it's compassion, it's feeling like we're in this together. Yeah, which is the same thing I felt when I met my wife, right? I'm actually married to a swami.

This is what it's all about. But I think that was the point of or that was the experience that I had. I don't know that it was a characteristic that other people saw in me so much, but my experience was that "Yeah, this is what life is about."

Somehow it just feels like it's evolved, it's just sort of more happened. I'm not a person who has sort of planned, okay, well, if I've got this, I should do this. This is what I want to do in five or ten years. I know I want to help people.

I think one of the other fascinating things about yoga was that there was this language that said what we do for others is really, really important. The lengths of common yoga, it's sort of where I believed but I never really knew how to talk about it before.

So I think that when you talk about what came along to help me to move forward, this was the recognition of giving back is the right thing to do. I have a hard time with the wording around that. But it is about sharing with others. As much as it's about receiving from others, it's about giving out.

I think another thing, it was the people. It's interesting as a physical therapist because sometimes people at the end of treatment would be so exuberant with their thanks.

Really, what I learned over time was saying to people, it's really not about me, it's about "You're the one that's done the work here." I've guided you and you have done the work. It's funny, this happened a few years ago; this one woman just touched my arm, and when I said that and she says, "Yeah, you'll figure it out." Or something like that, right?

It was something that at the time I didn't think a lot of because there was another patient coming in, but then it struck me later, it's like I've been so wrong about this. It is about me, right? So yes, the person has done the work, but what this person is telling me is that for whatever it was, yes, they know they did the work but there was something about me and the way that I worked with them.

I'm not specifically saying me, as in individual, as in my ego, there's something I was able to offer to them that actually allowed them to succeed where they hadn't been able to succeed before.

I really don't think that that's something, like I said, I don't think that that's something unique to me. I really think it has more to do with the love piece again.

The one other thing around this is that one of the things when I was teaching therapeutic yoga classes, I had people coming up to me, and this happened a bunch of times, people saying, "You know before I came here, I was in physical therapy and I was always trying to get better, I was trying to get better. What I found here is peace. You've offered me a place where I feel found, a place to stop fighting so much, stop struggling so much and I found that sense of peace."

To me each of those things sort of fits together, what was I able to, what people see in me or what was I able to offer them. Somehow, I was able to offer them a sense of hope and optimism and validation and empowerment and all those things that are so important once we start to practice yoga or the contemporary thing.

I also think to be able to do that we need to know how to hold space. We need to have some experience that really lands hard or lands well, and completely this idea that it is not our job to fix other people.

It's not our job always to fix a thing that's going on. It's not our job to offer that. Our job is to just really to hold space. Be there to listen to what the person is saying and then work with someone in the end to find the solution.

I think that a big part of my evolution is to be there, right? I think that's difficult definitely in terms of the yoga therapy, right? We want to be the expert; we want to be the person who's going to lead the person forward.

Practically, I would say as leaders and yoga therapists, we need to learn to sit at the feet of this other person, whether patient, client or whatever name we're giving, right?

We need to sit at their feet, they're the expert, and we also need to be in a place where they're sitting at our feet and we're okay with that. We also need to be in that place where we are colleagues, brainstormers, co-workers together.

I think in terms of leadership, I think this is the thing that's often missing when I think of how I was taught, because I was taught that I'm the expert, I have this knowledge, you don't have it, so I'm always here.

I think that's another thing that people have seen in me and I think that it's something that I've learned over a long period of time in this process of succeeding when things are complex.

The whole idea if you want to talk about yoga making us more flexible, to me that word should be more just this idea of adaptable and the importance of being able to adapt to the person that we're with to be able to serve them best. Because we can serve them best in many different ways. But most of us are taught that we always need to be this particular way.

As in the patient-centered goal setting that I hear people talking about, which teaches a lot of people that you are always there. Unfortunately, people get taught that rather than recognizing that it's the same, that's just one of the ways to do this.

But you still have expertise that the yoga person doesn't have. They may have expertise that you don't have. So it's not just being there; it's this—it's almost like physiological resilience, right?

We are healthy when things can vary up and down a lot.

I think as leaders we are most effective when we can morph to the situation that's happening in front of us rather than being the same all the time.

I've got a sense of it. I've been thinking about it a lot. It's the idea of really "Where do I go from here?" To me, there's a couple options. There's the option of just continuing on doing what I'm doing and the people who are interested in the work that I do around pain care and yoga...just keep on letting people know that I'm here and then they could come whether it's virtual or whether it's actually they come and do it in person.

That's what I really like to do, right? And they continue to share out, right? But there's this other thing of "Do I work on growing this because I think it's so important?" Do I actually take it, decide that my task is to try to take it in the works of the world, which is...I still don't know if that's the right path to take, which is interesting because I guess in terms of up until now I would say everything has been more of an evolution than a making a decision of what path I would take next.

I actually feel at this point that I sort of need to make a decision because the thing that would serve me the best would be to stop; it would be to not struggle, not to fight around this, not try to push.

I've done, within the physiotherapy world in Canada, I think that

I've done a lot to change the physiotherapy world around pain and pain care and science. So there's this "Do I want to step into that same thing?"

Do I want to step in and continue to try to push this or would it serve me more to step back and just see patients on my own here and just on my own? I just don't know which direction.

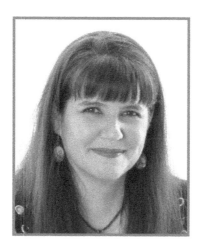

• • ● • •

Rose Kress, Owner and Director of LifeForce Yoga, and author, took her first yoga class in 1994. She began studying with Amy Weintraub in 2002, and in 2016, she purchased LifeForce Yoga from Amy. Rose developed a yoga therapy protocol for veterans and active duty soldiers receiving treatment for substance abuse and PTSD at a VA Health Care Center in Tucson, Arizona.

Rose creates online courses which make LifeForce Yoga more accessible. She is the creator of the Best Practices Series, a number of CDs/mp3s, including *Mantra Chanting with Rose*, *Yoga Nidra for Light and Clarity* and *True Heart Yoga Nidra*, and several LifeForce Yoga videos. In 2020, Rose published her first book, *Awakening Your Inner Radiance with LifeForce Yoga: Strategies for Coping with Depression, Anxiety, and Trauma*.

Rose Kress

Ihave no choice but to be working with people therapeutically with this understanding that yoga itself is not healing and I am not a healer of other people. I am a healer of myself; this is the tool, the technique that I use when working with others to give them the power to make these significant changes within themselves. And they make long-lasting changes within themselves.

Starting down this path of yoga, it's always been about healing. I knew from a very young age that I was supposed to be serving others in the healing capacity.

That was to be my pathway, innate, coming into the world with that. In 2004, I'd done yoga for years, I was in a program in Taiwan in a monastery and we were learning about monastic life, humanistic Buddhist monastic life.

We were in an ashram and meditating, Pure Land Buddhism mixed with Chan Buddhism. We were doing tai chi or kung fu and I was doing some yoga myself. I remember I taught one of the nuns yoga in one of the places, and then participants in the program said, "Hey, since you do so much yoga, you should teach us."

So they got me a room and I taught a yoga class in the room. It was the first time I think I really felt purely me. I wasn't nervous per se—I trained as a classical pianist, so I'm used to being open. I just let it flow.

It was in that moment where it's like "Oh my gosh, this is it. This is what I want to do, this is what I want to teach."

That was really the big shove to get me on that path.

Concurrently, my regular practice was with Amy Weintraub at a gym in Tucson, and she was always talking about depression. I had a really severe depressive episode, so I got that. I had really bad anxiety, but I wasn't really thinking of that as a pathway.

Amy said, "Oh, hey, I'm doing this training coming up—my first yoga for depression and anxiety. Do you want to help me with it?"

That moment was such an organic movement forward in terms of the trajectory with what I do, with the emotions and what I do with the mind. It is really the gift of past lifetimes, the gifts of healing, and for whatever reason, this coming in with knowledge of "This is what I'm supposed to be doing in my life with others." And there is a deep healing that needs to happen within myself. All of this training has, a lot of it, the physicality of yoga has been around managing my own physical issues and uniquely preparing me for future damages, which has been really interesting.

The Yoga Sutras say the only pain that can be prevented is that which is yet to come.

While I was not able to prevent pain from accidents, I was actually uniquely prepared to support myself through those major issues, concussions and neck injuries, in a way that I think a lot of people are not able to handle themselves.

One of the things I learned during my process is that I'm kinesthetic, and so I really operate from a place of feeling first. Then everything has to be translated, and it has to be translated into words, into imagery and into communication, and even into a thought process. Because operating from feeling states, there's not a thought process to it, it's just like "Just do it, because you just do it, because this is what my body is telling me to do."

With that in mind, in those teaching moments, I would have these resonances. Resonating experiences where I could see somebody doing something and I could feel within my body what was needed to counter it, to support readjustment. I call it my Jedi sense now; my Jedi skills have been honed, so I can see things going on in a different way.

The beginning stage, this understanding of myself of "Yes, yoga is the pathway, and here's how I can support people in moving this energy," was then coupled with what we would call a vasana in the Yoga Sutras, a pattern of behavior brought forward from previous lifetimes.

This vasana for me is the vasana of yoga wisdom, and all the yoga wisdom that is there.

I couldn't remember parts of the body after I had my concussion, I couldn't remember what to call...I'd be tapping my leg and looking for the word for leg. But I could remember the Yoga Sutras and these intense Sanskrit words and names for the poses. I couldn't remember any of the names of the poses in English, but I could remember them all in Sanskrit, which really spoke to me on a deep level; this is rooted within me in ways that I don't know how to speak to yet and that we may not understand in that Western methodology.

I was coming from this place of knowing that I'm supposed to be working with others and serving others, supporting them to heal themselves. The body's going to be my journey to do that and yoga is going to be the lens. I had gone to school for social work and I changed, like "Nope. I'm going to do this yoga thing instead." A lot of support and direction came always from teachers and colleagues and cohorts.

Of course, Amy was really instrumental in directing me down the emotional pathway to use yoga for supporting people with emotional upset, depression and anxiety. Then there was my other teacher, Maria Mendola, a phenomenal yoga therapy teacher. I was lucky enough to have her as one of my teacher trainers in my initial teacher training program. So I got a lot; within her, I saw a mind like mine with this capacity for remembrance of body and application of things.

My current teacher is Rama Jyoti Vernon, who just demonstrated an absolute trust and belief in me as an instructor.

I learned from her really that...I want to say the audacity to have complete confidence within myself as a gift from Rama, because if she trusts me and I trust her, then she sees something within me that maybe I don't. Maybe I'm believing those constrictive thought patterns that have been established in my life, and she sees that I can do this. If I trust her explicitly, that means I have to trust myself explicitly.

There were many other comments and support from friends and from my husband along the way, but those three gifts—the Magi, the three gifts of the Magi—those were really important gifts for me in moments of mistrust. Those gifts remain; yes, the essence of those gifts remains.

I'm just going to try this and see what happens. I was told, "You're really good at working with beginners, and you're really good at teaching gentle yoga, which is not easy to come out of a teacher training and be able to do that."

I kind of just went with that and was doing these very generic gentle yoga classes all at the gym and subbing here and there, but needing to bring in the practices.

Those things started coming in, and then sometimes they would come in the form of the body. When I met Rama in 2007, I'd been teaching for about two years at that point, I had this very confusing experience with breath a week beforehand. Here, this woman's about to come into your life, so you need to understand the depth of how the breath really works to fully be able to appreciate what you're about to do with this woman. That was the gift of back breathing and spinal extension in the exhale.

Through that experience, I shifted my language in therapeutic yoga classes. Bringing in language about the back and helping the back heal and helping to strengthen the back. One of my students was a chiropractor, and she would drop these little nuggets about what was happening with the body when we were doing these breathing practices.

That restructuring awareness and bringing awareness to deeper understandings of the body was met with a lot of resistance. There was a time for many years where I did not teach in a yoga studio at all. I was teaching for staff at the VA, I was teaching in a pulmonary office,

I was teaching in a hospital, a number of hospitals, I was teaching at a chiropractor's office, and not in a yoga studio.

The people that I am best suited to working with are people who have no understanding of the body, who don't feel their bodies, but need some sort of relief. I can bring them to those places because I've got that vasana of yoga in my energetics and in my life. I've got this understanding of the body.

My communication skills come from the person that I'm working with and from the person in front of me. If English is your second language and your vocabulary is 1000 words, I find myself speaking to you in a way where we're only using those 1000 words. If I am introducing a new word, I'm telling you what that word means. Or I worked with a blind woman once, so we have no visual aspects, so here's how I'm going to teach this. Or I taught in Spanish before to people, with my limited Spanish vocabulary, which is probably 1000, 2000 words.

It's really that awareness of understanding what my strengths are as a teacher, and as a person. What my worth is, and who is best suited to receive that support in the world. So yoga studios, there's a place for that, but non-yoga people—that's really the meat, that's really the juice.

The other way of knowing starts first with being with yourself. I know these things about myself, because, first, I spent all my time in this, I spend all my time with me. There are other people, but I do spend a lot of time alone. Because my body is so communicative, because I'm so kinesthetic, body often overrides thought process. I could be in a thought process, or I could be in a knowing, like "Oh yeah, this is what's supposed to happen here." My body speaks out to me.

Because that then leads to this co-creation, and if I know how to listen to myself—the signs and symbols being presented to me by a person in front of me, the universe, the trans-dimensional beings that are around me, the energy, whatever—if I can be around it and present within myself, then I have the capacity to hear that.

Some days, I'm 100 percent present and the ego is not there, and that information is flowing through. We are co-creating the practice together. Other days, and I'd say most of the time, 75 percent present, which I think is a really good number to be aiming for. I think 25 percent distraction, that's okay. But that 75 percent—that's the goal.

For me, confidence is this sense of trusting myself. Not trusting that I know what's right or I know what's wrong, or I know a piece of information, because all of that is constantly changing.

That's why there's been this "*me to we*" trajectory. I'm confident in my ability to listen to what's coming forward, and that whatever is arising and coming forward is something to follow, and that there is wisdom there.

In terms of creating things, right now, particularly with COVID and the quarantine, there's been this sense that everything needs to change. I'm going to say as well that there has been this: we've been on a trajectory and things need to change. We can't keep doing things the way they are, and it's not working. I've been saying for years the yoga studio model is dead, it's just dead. It's not really working the way it once worked, if it ever worked. The way we're behaving environmentally in the world is dead; it needs to change. It's killing us, it's literally killing us.

So here we are with this virus that has forced us to step back and to stay home, and there's been this grieving process of "I can't do things the way that I have been doing things, and I'm being forced into a change."

This sense of creating needs to cease for a moment, and it did, and it's been shifting now into this sense of greater creativity. The darkness in the world, it literally...it does an action and that action has a lot of growth around it.

We must ask each other, "What are you creating and bringing forth into the world, and how are you creating that and how does that serve this sense of light coming together?"

That has started to shift into "What do people need right now? What am I sharing for people about what they need? How can I now bring that into...?" and it's congealing into some online course work of life skills.

Because as yoga skills, as life skills—because what am I seeing and hearing from people so much? A significant lack of life skills.

I can teach you how to manage your sadness, your grief, so that you can move forward.

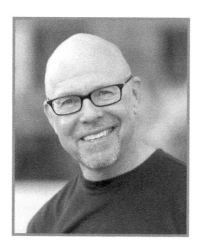

• • • • •

Stephen Cope is a best-selling author and scholar who specializes in the relationship between the Eastern contemplative traditions and Western depth psychology. Publications include *Yoga and the Quest for the True Self*, *The Wisdom of Yoga* and *The Great Work of Your Life*. His most recent work, *Deep Human Connection*, is an examination of the psychology, neurobiology and spirituality of deep human connection, and the imperatives of human attachment.

Stephen has been Scholar-in-Residence at the Kripalu Center for Yoga and Health for nearly 30 years, the largest center for the study and practice of yoga in the Western world, located in Stockbridge, Massachusetts. Stephen is the founder and former director of the Kripalu Institute for Extraordinary Living, a research institute examining the effects and mechanisms of yoga and meditation, with a broad team of researchers.

In its 25th anniversary edition, *Yoga Journal* named Stephen one of the most influential thinkers, writers and teachers on the current American yoga scene.

Stephen Cope

When I was back in the old ashram days, we had a beloved member of the ashram who was dying of AIDS at that time. There was a care team that I was part of because I was a close friend of his. As he slowly died, I remember his taking my hand one day and saying to me, "Kavi, I have to tell you something that I've learned as I've been dying. The only skill, finally, that you can take out with you is the capacity to surrender, so learn that lesson well and practice surrendering and letting go." That's the phase I'm in, and it's quite marvelous. Because it's rather like being in psychoanalysis, where you learn this deep profound trust. The Chinese put it as, "It's trust in mind, the great form of trust in mind is all about that lesson." The Tao Te Ching is all about that lesson. Those are some of the things that I look at now, during this phase of surrender.

I was on fire with the dharma.

I recognized it. I was on fire with its empiricism, with its subtlety, with its genius. I'll never forget, that summer; I was completely on fire for the dharma, and I really dropped in. Eventually, the center moved out to Newton, and I went with it. They say that it was, like back in the 1970s, when this happened, that you could meet your guru in Harvard Square. In fact, that's where I was. I did meet Chögyam Trungpa Rinpoche and his group of crazy wisdom people there.

Every day, I'd look at that scene and I thought, "What are they doing?" Because I really didn't know what meditation was. One day, I just boldly walked in and said to the guy, "What are you doing?" He said, "We're studying meditation. Would you like to join us?"

I was open. It's one of the things I remember about my early days in this world. I was so open to everything. Who isn't? One of the great writers says that in order to explore this world, you need three things. You need openness, skepticism and common sense.

It's funny, because I'd never heard about Shakti. I had no idea that it was possible. It wasn't something I made up in my head. I didn't even know what it was until later. That sealed the deal. I was going to go to Kripalu. It took me an entire year to detach from my psychoanalytic, psychotherapy practice. I had lots of long-term clients. I remember the very day when I was sitting in my apartment in Jamaica Plain, praying about this. I prayed about it a lot. The more I practiced, the more I found that there was this still, small voice, this inner voice. The Christians call it the still, small voice, this knowing. I was sitting, meditating in my living room, and it was the closest thing to actually hearing a voice that my still, small voice has ever produced, which said, "You will take a year off and you will investigate this. You must."

In those days, there were 350 of us running around at Kripalu. We had this totally live guru. We had Satsang every night. Satsang is at the feet of the guru, and with lots of instruments and crazy, wild dancing. It was a full-on ashram experience that I had there for five years. I like to call it now the reparative family experience because it was like a big family in the living room. I don't know if you were there in those days, but Satsang at night was wild and crazy. We worked 60 hours a week doing seva. I had five years of a truly amazing reparative family experience there, where I was valued and seen and mirrored. I became a valuable part of the community and so I bloomed. I was really in it. I was in the belly of the beast.

I remember my first book because I had lived this dream fantasy world of Kripalu in its heyday, at its very best. All of us who are old-timers and spent 30 years there talk about it as a miraculous time that we were so lucky to have. As you know and as most readers will probably know, it fell apart in 1994; that was after I'd been there for five years, when the guru was having inappropriate relationships with students, so our community asked him to leave. When that happened, it was a huge scandal.

My friends and all of the senior students had decided it was our dharma to translate this ashram experience into a more mainstream experience into which we could enlighten everyone. We had this building which would house 500 people. It was a gift, and it was a dharma and it was a sacred duty. I can't believe that it fell into my lap and I'm not sure where I got the balls to do it, but I did it. That was the beginning of my writing career, and I've been writing ever since. I'm right now working on my sixth book.

We sketched it all out that night, huddling in a corner. Over the next ten years, we would make it real. The idea was to make yoga accessible, viable and acceptable in a world based on science. We needed to investigate the effects, the mechanisms, the dosing and everything else about yoga. That's the next task for anybody who's interested in moving this out into the larger world. We knew that we wanted to move yoga into the healthcare system and the educational system, and that in order to do that we would have to have our scientific bona fides in a row. We started with nothing. We raised a lot of money. I would have to say, millions of dollars over those nine years that I directed the Kripalu Institute for Extraordinary Living.

The only thing that comes into my mind is this book is driven by what's true. What do I know that's true? What do I have to say that's true?

That's it.

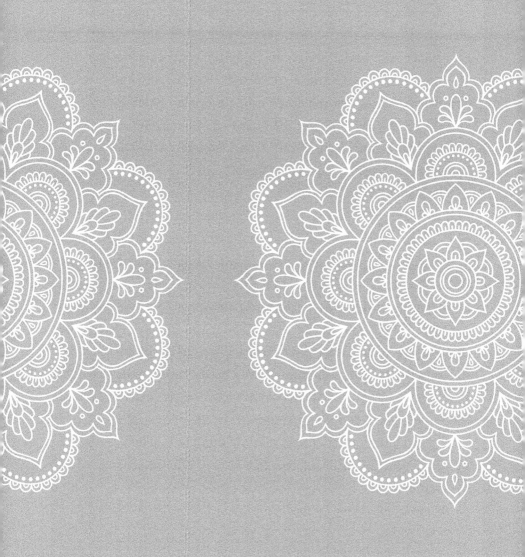

VII

Further Reflections

*Listening to the universe with
others, listening again.*

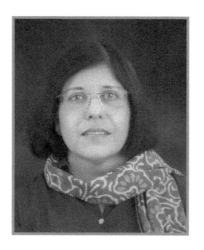

• • ● • •

Shirley Telles has a degree in conventional medicine (MBBS) and an MPhil and PhD in Neurophysiology. Both MPhil and PhD theses were on the effects of yoga practice. Dr. Telles received a Fulbright fellowship in 1998 and in 2001 an award from the Templeton Foundation for creative ideas in neurobiology. In 2007, supported by the Indian Council of Medical Research Center for Advanced Research, she piloted research to study meditation's effects through autonomic variables, evoked and event-related potentials, polysomnography and fMRI. Since 2007, Dr Telles has been the director of Patanjali Research Foundation, Haridwar, India. She has more than 198 research papers cited in bibliographic databases and has authored seven books.

Shirley Telles

My way of functioning is rather different from what most people would imagine, the way most people function. Mine is very unplanned, and if anything occurs to me to be done, it's usually an impulse, and with the passion, and until it sees friction, until it's realized, I don't have any peace. I mean, I'm really spilling over with energy until I get it done. Because it's something that is just wound up in me like passion or an excitement.

It's not a very thinking thing.

When I joined here, I just knew that I wanted to study the brain, and I didn't want to study rats and monkeys, and I don't like dissecting animals. I wanted to do human studies. Then the person who guided me gave me a number of options, and said, "Maybe you can look at everything that's going on and all our projects, see what you'd like to do."

One project was on the effect of malnutrition and how it affects the brain. I didn't really like that. I wanted to study sleep. I was very fascinated by sleep. But then the person who guided me said, "I somehow feel that the area which has a lot of future is yoga."

I didn't know anything about yoga in 1988 and I was fresh from medical college, and I felt it was a lot of nonsense. Then I happened to mention it at home, and my mother said, "I really think you should take this up." She still loves yoga, and she's very happy that I've done it. She had a book, and I had read the book as a child too, but it didn't make any impact on me. She said, "I've always practiced some form of yoga in my life." Even though I listen to my mother quite a bit, I would say that's been quite a guiding, a source of inspiration for me, but we don't always agree, but I really believe that something coming from her has worth.

I also valued my guide. Was a very sensible person. At first, I was very angry that I was being given this nonsensical topic. But then it gradually shifted to interest. I was given a whole lot of books to read by my guide, a whole stack—really a pile. I went back and read them, and I was still not convinced. Then one person from Bangalore who I'm still very much in contact with led a class. For the first time, at the end of the class, I could feel a difference. I should give you the background.

At this time, when I was entering into the study, I used to get very anxious. I used to easily go into panic attacks. It looked like asthma, but it was not. Particularly, if I had a deadline, or exam, I used to really get into the spiral and often needed a bronchodilator.

But it wasn't an asthmatic attack. Many people were puzzled what it was. Then I could feel this sort of quietening as I practiced for the first 45 minutes, and it sort of caught my interest. I said, "I want another session." I did have another session. We all did. There were a whole lot of people practicing along with me. Then that's when I really decided this is what I want to take up. It was very difficult at the time, because most of the other people in that institute thought it was a ridiculous thing. They thought you should study, they would say, "It's an institute of mental health and neurosciences!" No one else was studying yoga, and they said it's a very foolish thing to take up.

Of course, it's very interesting that now, more than 30 years later, that institute is very actively engaged in yoga research. That's how it started for me.

A lot of the first important meetings I had were recommended by my guide, and they're the people I'm in contact with even today. I was in a stage of exploration; completed two years, so it was very cerebral at that stage. It wasn't a hard journey, and then I was entering my doctoral stage. I still had thoughts of shifting my topic, and looking at single neurons, and what are the changes during specific activities, and so on. Then my guide said, "Still, I think you have really done a nice job already in yoga, why don't you think of doing your PhD in this area?" I wasn't opposed to it anymore, but I was not yet enthusiastic. Then my guide said to me, "There is a brother and sister, very simple, they are very focused and very academic. Maybe you'd like to meet them. You may have heard of them. Dr. Nagudna, and Dr. Nagendra from Bangalore."

I met them, and they really helped me for my PhD. I think for the first time I saw academicians. She's a doctor and very focused. Her brother, Dr. Nagendra, is MD PhD. I could see that though the degrees were in conventional education, they had really gotten into yoga. They're living a yoga life. Gradually, I started going more to the center, which was like an ashram, then spending time in the institute. I think that's where I landed.

Not only in this center, which I've mentioned, but even in others like, there's a center for Raga Yoga meditation, which was the topic for my PhD. I really used to spend time there and learned the meditation. I used to go there at 4:30 in the morning—that's a very different space, very different. Then I really enjoyed it, and there was no looking back after that.

At every stage door, I always trust many people, like I first observe people critically, and then I decide if I trust them or not. But even then, I have a lot of internal inquiry, internal chatting, and only after that is over, and a lot of it goes on, then I listen from the heart, as well from the brain, and then I say yes, I can go with what so-and-so is saying.

For me, it's always a combination. I can't give the percentages. It's a combination of critical analysis and observation. For example, I think this is very important, because we see this a lot in the yoga world, so it's not just enough to trust.

You have to really critically analyze and continuously reappraise and think, "Is it all right to trust this person or not? Is the person worthy of my trust? Are their actions and are their words and deeds compatible? Do they say something? Do they do the same thing, or do they do something completely off the mark?" I would say that even some of the people who I—none of the people that I mentioned, but further along when I did trust them, and used the wisdom—I could also see that there were certain gaps between what they suggested and what they did. It wouldn't be total trust.

I think that's a very important part. You should be able to see the person who's giving you the wisdom for what they are. You should not be blinded to the quality, thinking that they are all-knowing or all-giving, whatever. No one is. We should always see someone as a human being. That, I feel, is most critical.

First thing I would say is that I always have a very strong saying for myself, that whenever you do something, you should make an informed decision, give it your absolute best. I mean, you don't compromise in your effort. Then, whatever is the outcome, it's in a way like my yoga, you should be comfortable with it. This has been my thing right from the beginning. I used to edit a school magazine when I was very young. I put this into one of the editions, and one of my friends remembered it. She said, "Oh, you've written this." That's really my bottom line.

But I would also add that I really don't know; I would say this because it is important to me: I link it with my faith in God.

It's very important to me. Once I believe that I have made a decision, and I'm giving it my best, there's no compromise in my principles, then whatever comes of it, I accept happily.

In Karma Yoga, we have a very strong idea about how we should be. You cannot be bothered by the fruits of your action; it's a good wave. It's a sort of control, or it's a nice way of regulating our behavior and the way we work. But there are times when we should allow the real self to function without these boundaries. I think if you're developing in the yoga part, you will fit within the Karma Yoga framework but in a spontaneous way. It would be just bubbling through you. And without being consciously aware that you are not worried about the fruits of your action, or you're not doing it for a particular endpoint, the endpoint is seeing the task completed. The endpoint is not seeing a particular result or getting a particular gratification.

Raga Yoga is again very systematic. Because it is the eight steps. It is also planned. You go through the yamas, niyamas, you consciously make a decision that you want to reach a particular point. Yamas, niyamas, you observe them, and you go through your body culturing with asana, then pranayama, pratyahara, then very much so, mental control, in dharana, regulating attention. Until the dharana phase, you don't leave the focus. It's only in dhyana and samadhi that you let go. I would say that the spontaneity can only come out of the parts in Bhakti Yoga. That's where the cortex is dampened, and it's entirely from the sub-cortical level that one is functioning in a very regulated way.

Yes, I think that one of the reasons people choose community is to try to do deep practices. Of course, unfortunately, it may not always be safe. But the basic premise is that these kinds of communities are safe. I would say that the majority of them, if critically evaluated and a person doesn't lose their senses, and lives in the community sensibly, they are safe. Unlike the prevailing norm that people think that it is unsafe outside, if it is safe, definitely, it creates a sort of situation. Obviously, when you feel safe, you have less sympathetic arousal. When you have less sympathetic arousal, your attention, orienting, alerting, responses, and certain parts of the cortex which are involved in that, can shut down. When they can shut down, and the blood is not required then—a very crude way of saying it—it can be diverted to other parts of the brain which have the potential to maybe allow us to be more creative, more explorative, I would say.

I mean, that's the time you really go inwards and understand yourself. That's only possible if you feel safe. You can reach that level of gratitude and self-exploration only when you really feel you don't have any immediate needs, and worries, and you feel you're in a protected space.

If there is something that I would say spontaneously lives with me and continues to inspire me, I will always say to whoever, whenever I'm talking about my journey in yoga, just one thing, that every person should choose. "If you're convinced you want to do something, whatever it is, you should do it in a way that makes every single day, and every part of the day that you're working or doing that thing, that it is enjoyable." That's the only thing I would say. That every day, you should approach your activity with the same amount of excitement, freshness and enjoyment. That's all. It should be irrespective of the monetary remuneration, or what you're otherwise going to get from it, nothing matters. I really say this passionately, because in the start of my career, I was actually working free for quite some time.

Yes, so I mean it's exciting to be alive, I think.

Excitement just to be.

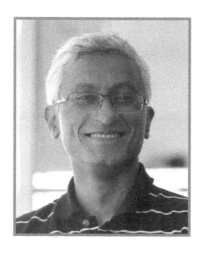

• • ● • •

Ganesh Mohan is the son of A.G. Mohan and Indra Mohan, practicing yoga from childhood. Trained in both modern medicine and Ayurveda, his work focuses on the application of yoga for health and wellbeing in chronic health conditions and lifestyle diseases. He developed the Svastha Yoga Therapy Program in 2010 and serves as advisor and presenter to many international yoga training organizations and conferences. The Mohan family continues to be active in training yoga teachers with a focus on therapeutic and individualized work. Publications include *Yoga Therapy* (Shambhala Publications, 2004), *Krishnamacharya: His Life and Teachings* (Shambhala Publications, 2010), *Yoga Reminder: Lightened Reflections* (Svastha Yoga, 2015), *Yoga Yajnavalkya* (Svastha Yoga, 2013) and *Hatha Yoga Pradipika* (Svastha Yoga, 2017).

Ganesh Mohan

There is a lot to be absorbed from the wisdom of some traditional systems. Being a bridge between older systems and what we're doing in modern times now, more structured learning approaches, is really one of my most important goals. To make sure that it's done with fairness, a sense of community, with integrity and depth. These are all values that I'm sure all of us would aspire to, right?

I learned yoga without ever realizing because my parents started teaching yoga even before I was born. My father always used to say that it is not necessary to become a yoga teacher, but it is essential to practice yoga. It was not my intention to become a yoga teacher. It just happened that I found that there was meaning in what I learned when I was young. What I always wanted to be was a doctor, which is what I ended up becoming. And then by the time I completed my medical studies, I had already studied Ayurveda. And by the time I completed my medical studies, I realized that I didn't want just to be another doctor.

That has been one of my major drivers—to see what I can take from the ancient sources, which I seem to have observed quite a lot of without even realizing. I studied Sanskrit formally when I was young. I studied Ayurveda privately with my teacher who's more than 85 years old now. And I used to study every day and see patients with him. My experience of learning was very different from many current Western adaptations. The traditional system of learning was not about asking what are the competencies I'm going to learn? You start with a text and you sit with your teacher, and then you learn little by little as time goes on. It's a commitment of seven years.

Samkhya and yoga and Ayurveda assume that the sense of self is what creates the world. That from my sense of self comes my subjective world. And what is an objective world? I guess just different subjective worlds that we agree upon. If you and I both agree on the same thing, then they say it is objective. But, ultimately, each one of us is coming from only our own subjective perspective.

There will be different ways of looking at the sense of self that is frozen into all these systems that derive from there. Consequently, I think a there are a lot of the aspects of co-creation that we would like to move towards nowadays, that don't try to manipulate the environment, that don't try to manipulate other living beings. We can co-create the state of wellbeing by acknowledging that we are interdependent. We are connected and that cannot be separated in any meaningful way whatsoever. In fact, if you were to choose to separate any or all of these things, we would not exist in the way we already are.

That foundational shift, however, has to also exist with some degree of structure.

When the Yoga Sutra talks about asana, pranayama, the eight limbs of yoga, yama, niyama, asana, pranayama, pratyahara, dharana, dhyana, samadhi, the commentaries point out that the ultimate state of samadhi comes about only when all the limbs co-exist. They are like spokes of a wheel. There are also steps in a sense. The commentaries point out both. There is some progression of structure involved, yet you cannot separate them. You cannot understand thinking without the body, it's a bit of the same thing, like asking: What is a feeling? Without the senses, what is a feeling? Without the breath, what is a feeling?

This apparent conflict between structure and organic systems is profoundly interesting. And that is not a new conflict, actually. You can look back, I think, at more ancient systems of learning. We find that they developed ways of creating structure that are perhaps a lot more realistic and reflect the reality of the world much better.

Uncertainty is built into the nature of the universe. Chaos is the word that we use. Now, chaos is also a form of creativity. The more we try to structure everything, the more we lose the infinite possibilities that the universe provides. From the perspective of yoga, the Bhagavad Gita instructs that the pathway of karma is deep and invisible. Why do you exist as a human being now? Yoga's point is that it is your karma. Now, you may think of it from a medicine or a metaphysical perspective, yet it is interesting to contemplate that our physical reality is a manifestation of the unconscious tendencies that your consciousness manifests.

When we become embodied, our samskaras, our unconscious, is infinite. The potential is infinite.

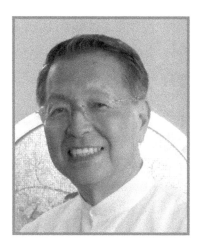

• • ● • •

Kazuo Keishin Kimura founded the Japan Yoga Therapy Society and is the Society's President. In 2019, he was invited by World Health Organization (WHO) Traditional, Complementary and Integrative Medicine as one of 20 international experts to attend the WHO Working Group Meeting on Benchmarks for Training in Yoga. He is currently engaged in activities to promote traditional yoga and yoga therapy in Japan, India, Europe and North and South America. His newest book in English, *India's 5000-Year-Old Psychotherapy: Yoga Therapy Darshana*, is scheduled to be published in summer 2021.

Kazuo Keishin Kimura

At that time, I realized that traditional yoga exercises and the yoga therapy exercises I had learned before were quite different. When I met my guru for first time, he asked me why I came to Yoga Niketan. It was during what we call darshana—to meet a guru. I told him my aim was to reach the final state of mind. He said, "OK, I accept you."

So you know, now I am 74, but when I was a college student in Tokyo, many young Americans came to Japan to escape the draft for the Vietnam War. Europe was unstable too, and I didn't have much hope for society. I thought if I studied science, I might at least contribute something, but my science professors did not give us hope either. So I transferred to study religious philosophy at Kyoto University for two years.

I talked to a professor at Kyoto University about my future. He was a Buddhist monk, and he recommended against reading philosophy. I think he wanted me to enter a Buddhist monastery, but I was not interested, because the lives of modern monks are actually not very spiritual. But his recommendation to engage in spiritual practice left an impression.

After completing my studies, I moved to my wife's home town near the Japan Sea. I had no idea how to do spiritual practices and started fishing. A couple years later, I had a chance to go to Europe for a wedding, and decided to travel overland to India after that. I traveled by land through Germany, Turkey, Iran and Afghanistan, and finally reached India. That was 1974.

There was not much information about yoga then, but I found the Kaivalyadhama Yoga Institute in Lonavala. They had a one-year college program to study a therapeutic type of yoga. I attended, but I had wanted to meet traditional yogis and practice traditional yoga.

They had a yogic hospital there, and one day a Belgian woman came to the hospital suffering from asthma. I ended up taking care of her when she had a severe asthmatic attack at midnight. I helped her through her attack, and then while she was resting, I looked at some of her books. One had intriguing pictures, so I asked her who the author was. She said the author was her guru in the Himalayas, and that in the winter, he comes down from the mountains to Rishikesh. It was winter at that time, so I took a train to Rishikesh, and this is how I met my guru.

I stayed with my guru for about one month and meditated with him in the meditation hall in Rishikesh. He founded an ashram there, Yoga Niketan. I'm Japanese, so I knew about Zen meditation, but I went to India to learn traditional Indian meditation.

I wanted to find a solution to bring people happiness. So I followed my guru, Swami Yogeshwaranada Maharaj, for ten years in the Himalayas. I took Guru Dīkṣā, an initiation ceremony, at Yoga Niketan Rishkesh on March 3, 1982 at age 35, and I became his direct disciple. He gave me the name Jnana Yogi.

My guru knew the final wisdom which is called Atma Vijnana and Brahma Vijnana. He learned this traditional Raja yoga and its wisdom from an Indian guru living in Tibet near Mount Kalish, in a place called Tirta Puri.

After spending eight years with him, he told me to teach Raja yoga to other people. At first, I refused, but he did not accept that. He told me again, "You should teach Raja yoga." I didn't disagree after that, because I knew it was rude to say no to a superior person twice. This was the first time for me to shift my yoga practice, moving from "me" to "we."

So I started to teach Raja yoga to people in Japan. Many people approached me because I knew traditional yogic practices and had studied with my guru in the Himalayas for a long time. Many were yoga teachers, and some had hundreds of students. I taught them from among several hundred types of asanas, pranayama and meditation techniques. But sometimes they asked me how to teach yoga to pregnant women, patients with panic disorder, or students who had breast cancer surgery.

I had no idea how to teach yoga to people who were ill. I had stayed at a yoga therapy institute once, but they had no method to diagnose or treat patients through the yoga tradition. I told my Raja yoga students that I had no idea how to diagnose or treat such patients. But they continued to ask me. And when I learned that people with medical problems also continued to go to their yoga classes, even though the instructors didn't know how to handle them, I gradually changed my mind. I started investigating how I could help people suffering from various kinds of diseases. This was my second time to change myself from "*me*" to "*we*."

I realized that in yogic tradition, every time I met my guru, he assessed my mind and situation and then gave me instructions. My guru's education was not in medicine or clinical psychology, and yet he assessed and instructed each disciple.

To me, that meant he must have had a method to assess his disciples' body and mind. And he knew how to educate different kinds of pupils through yoga's tradition, wisdom and techniques. I started to guess what kinds of techniques and knowledge he used for assessment and instruction, based on all my experiences learning from him.

My guru taught me theories of human structure and function. They were the pancha kosha theory from the Taittiriya Upanishad, and the human chariot theory from the Katha Upanishad and Bhagavad Gita. I realized that they were yogic anatomy and physiology, used to understand human existence. My practice was to learn how to control the human chariot to overcome years of imbalance. That is the core of Raja yoga teachings.

Aside from Raja yoga education, I met a medical doctor from Bangalore when she visited Japan in October 1987. I learned that she was also using the pancha kosha model to treat her patients in their yoga therapy facility called Prashanti Kutiram.

I learned that they had many patients from all over the world. We discussed how to use Indian yogic wisdom to assess and treat patients. Eventually, they introduced me to two ways to propagate yoga therapy to society, and this was the third chance to change my mind from "*me*" to "*we*."

One recommendation was to collaborate with top researchers in Japan for yoga therapy research and gather evidence for yoga therapy.

The second is, teaching yoga to students, yoga teachers at the time could not explain the mechanism for why yoga works to promote health. So, in 1988, I started yoga therapist training courses all over Japan.

In 2014 we got a research grant from the government. We surveyed about 3000 yoga participants all over Japan. We asked about their conditions and their motivation to join yoga classes. We collected about 2500 valid responses, and more than 50 percent said they had chronic illnesses—mostly psychosomatic. More than 40 percent said they were receiving outpatient care while also attending yoga classes. That means the majority of yoga class participants have medical problems and their main motivation is to improve their health.

My son is a medical doctor and doctors are not lazy. But we know medicine is symptomatic treatment and doesn't cure the root causes of psychosomatic illnesses, which are in the mind. Some people have stomach ulcers, high blood pressure or diabetes mellitus, but medical doctors cannot treat the root causes if caused by mental disturbances. That's why the patients come to yoga. My wife is a clinical psychologist, but yoga class participants are also not satisfied with counseling because their symptoms are mainly somatic.

My guru had three gurus in his lifetime. One was a monk in his village temple. He met the second as a teenager, and he learned all the fundamental Raja yoga techniques, several hundred types of asanas and more than 100 pranayama and meditation techniques, some that required sitting for 24 hours without changing positions. He met his third guru when he was in his 50s near the source of Ganges. The third guru told my guru he would initiate him to the traditional wisdom of Atma Vijnana and Brahma Vijnana, but only if my guru promised not to hide in the Himalayas, but to go to town to teach people. My guru promised, and after being initiated, my guru stayed in a cave for three years, three months and three days without meeting anyone in order to make the wisdom firm in his mind. Then he came down to Gangotri and Rishikesh to teach spiritual seekers.

I understand my guru's story. My guru also told me to teach, so that is our fundamental motivation. Through the teachings of Raja yoga and yoga therapy, I now teach how to help people with health problems, using methods of assessment and instruction from the yoga tradition that I learned through transmission from my guru. People can buy my guru's book about Atmavijnana and Brahmavijnana from Yoga Niketan Delhi ashram, and I also sell my yoga therapy books on Amazon. But as you know, yoga wisdom cannot be gained only through reading books. Without practice, tapas and sadhana, we cannot reach such an ultimate state of mind.

Yoga pupils respect me because I practice the tradition, and I cooperate with medical researchers and clinical psychologists to establish methods of assessment and treatment. So from the yoga side it's okay, but some medical people don't trust us, and clinical psychologists feel some kind of envy, because they have no systematic theories of human structure and function like yoga does. But researchers of psychosomatic medicine are interested. We work closely with one such researcher at one of Japan's top national medical schools. Another is an advisor to the Japan Yoga Therapy Society. He introduced me to several medical researchers in Japan, and through them, we have been able to collaborate for research with grants from the Japanese government. This gives evidence that yoga therapy works. One research project was introduced on Harvard University School of Medicine's yoga homepage—the title is "Nationwide survey on adverse events of yoga." Another paper was awarded by the American scientific journal *Springer Nature* as one of their "Change the World, One Article at a Time" in 2018 in the field of medicine and public health.

One time, my guru told me that when he practiced Raja yoga in the Himalayas, in the dense forest, or deep in the Himalayan caves, his worries were resolved quite simply. His mind was liberated. But as I told you, his third guru told him to teach. So my guru started many programs, founded the ashram and wrote books, and many people approached him. He said that created disturbance in his mind, so his mind was not steady any more. [laughing] My guru told us that when he listened to troubles from other people, his mind also synchronized to the problem, making his mind very busy. But my guru was happy to help all the people. So this is a complicated matter when we go from the state of "*me*" to "*we*."

As I mentioned, there are two kinds of the highest wisdom in India. One is Atma Vijnana and the other one is Brahma Vijnana. Each Vijnana is relative wisdom, as "vi" in Sanskrit means "relative" in English. They mean wisdom of Atman and science of Brahman. And through these two, we have to reach perfect harmony with this universe, with nature, and people in society. Sage Patanjali called this wisdom viveka kyathi (awareness of the distinction between the Self and the not-Self), to know the perfect state of mind, "*we*." May all of us go to this "*we*" state of mind through yoga.

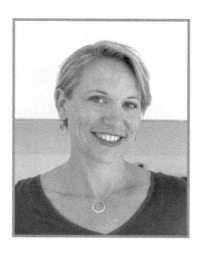

• • ● • •

Ann Marie Johnston is an entrepreneur, yoga teacher, marketing strategist and mom/mum of two. She is the founder and director of YogaMate, a digital healthtech platform with a mission of empowering people in their journey towards better health and wellbeing. Ann Marie is an invited guest lecturer on webinars within yoga therapy master's programs and yoga service leadership, alongside podcasts; she has also featured in national and international media.

In 2020, Ann Marie was awarded a Presidential Commendation from the IAYT (International Association of Yoga Therapists) and Give Back Yoga Foundation for conceiving, developing and producing the Global Yoga Therapy Day.

Ann Marie Johnston

I'm in union when I have those embodied responses that tell me, "Yes. You're on the right track." And I trusted that. And I try as much as possible to stop the head. The head is the thing that stops us from progress.

It kind of baffles me now, thinking back to it, that we could get to some 30 years of age and not even know that it was a possibility to stop this incessant chatter that is happening in our heads.

That it is majorly negative chatter. That it was the catalyst for change. Over the years, I dove more into a very personal practice, which is very centered and very meditative. There's very little physical. But that was the spark. And so I remember deciding in 2012 that I could see such clear transformation in my wellbeing.

And the only thing is yoga practice. I wanted to understand why my life has shifted so significantly, and how. I wanted my own personal understanding of why this practice had shifted my life so dramatically.

I had been melancholic, in a chronic depressive state since I was quite young. It just was my state of being. I had been taking depression medicine for seven years, and I had chronic headaches and irritable bowel syndrome and a really irregular menstrual cycle. Just really not in vibrant health. And one day, in conjunction with...it was the week and a half or so before I started my teacher training and I realized I am taking these pills every day mindlessly. Just because.

I found no point to life.

And I got to the halfway point (in my teacher training) and I thought, "It would be negligent of me to not share this." I remember distinctly where I was in the moment.

It was 2012. I said, "I can see myself working at a government level or something trying to get yoga more accessible to more people." Those were kind of my two moments. Like the first "aha" moment of "Holy crap, what have I been missing out my whole life on?" And a few years later when I made that decision, that I have to share this. This is too important. Everyone deserves this knowledge.

But then, conversely, I look out and I see this misperception that there is about what yoga is.

It's not just about the physical practice. I wanted people to understand that yoga is the breath. And it's meditation, and it's the connection to self, and it's the consciousness, right? I wanted to share that.

Everyone can do this practice; if you can breathe, you can do yoga.

And so it's interesting because I almost, in some ways, find—and this is years on—that it's hard to put the word yoga on it because people have this concept and this misperception of what yoga is. And it becomes so limited and narrow.

So, the original idea for YogaMate was about four months after I had finished my yoga teacher training. I had had my son. And I remember I was meditating one morning and suddenly it came into my mind that if the practice was just on my phone, then I wouldn't have to look for these sheets of paper every week, right?

And then it kind of went from there. If it was on my phone, then I could share it with my students, and they wouldn't be reliant on me to teach them all the time. They would be able to begin to develop their own personal practice.

And again, it was like, this needs to be on your phone. And so it kind of all coalesced, this idea around providing the practices in a digital, quick-access way.

And I thought, "That's a good idea. That's a good idea."

I reached back out to Leigh Blashki, and said, "Look, I understand that you're in retirement, but can you help me identify the individuals who should be part of this? Who can help me steer and guide this and take it forward?"

And he said, "No, no, no. I want to be involved."

So he gets involved. And that made the absolute world of difference, because he had the clout. He had the contacts. He had the relationships. And his stamp of approval opened up the doors for me to connect with some people who were very smart and willing.

I find that ideas come when you least expect them, right? So always be ready to write down the idea, because if you don't grab hold of it, it will be gone, and you can't act on it. So I used to keep a notepad next to my bed, so if I woke up in the middle of the night, I could jot something down. Or when I woke up in the mornings, I would reflect on any dreams that came to me or whatnot. Same with meditation. I would meditate on a question and then write anything that came to me. When an idea comes, I don't look at it through the lens of all the problems. I just look at it as "How do you get it done?"

But there are these inherent core values that are pulling from each of these, and we can pull that together.

So, I think the key there is that I have trusted that creative insight or impulse and often I'll get a shiver, I'll get a signal. A physical signal that I've hit a truth.

I'm in union when I have those embodied responses that tell me, "Yes. You're on the right track." And I trusted that. And I try as much as possible to stop the head. The head is the thing that stops us from progress.

And you learn to put it aside and just trust. Trust that what's come through to you has come to you for a reason and that you are positioned to make it work. And that somehow things will align in a way to execute this, and it might not look exactly as you picture it's going to be, but you also have to surrender and let go of what the outcome is going to be.

And I'm just going to allow and I'm going to release as much as I can what the results are, and trust that I've done what I was here to do.

Other like-minded individuals can help me take this beyond my limited resources and ways. January was when I was going to be kicking off the planning for Global Yoga Therapy Day 2020. And I can't do that right now. And so what does that mean? And it's my baby, and for the baby to flourish, I have to let the baby go. I have to hand the baby to someone else. My business just got put on the shelf. And the pure hassle of this corona timing thing!

I would feel grateful for being fulfilled. These past couple months have been very much a pause mode for me and now with the homeschooling and COVID stuff, it just still feels the pause is there. But again, I do feel it's beginning to shift and lift. My sense of purpose has been a bit rudderless, and for me, that has been very challenging. I feel like if everyone could come onboard with the same vision and work together and could move this stuff forward, I would feel very fulfilled personally that I have done what I'm here to do.

Hopefully, I am someone who is very centered and humble. And purposeful. Dedicated.

And yeah, there's this money thing that sits there, yet that's not why I'm here. I don't believe the framework of my society and my culture, my upbringing, my family and my ex-husband, yet obviously a very small unconscious part of me does still equate success to that.

And, basically, how can I trust in that? I think that, all of a sudden, the kids were with me fully and I couldn't focus on my business. How can I juggle both? How can I be a single mom with full-time kid care and still do this? And so I've been quiet. And then this COVID thing happened and I was like, "Oh, there's my excuse." I don't have to say, "I'm a single mom and it's been hard, and I've had my own personal stuff," because we don't need to go into that, but I can kind of lean on the fact that the world's changed.

And this gives me space for it to be okay that I have been quiet for a few months. And that was a permission that I was granting myself because I had these expectations of who I had to be.

I am courage. I love the concept of collaboration. Selfishness is not quite the right word, but like just coming from a space of giving. Like heartfelt desire for the good for everyone. Not help for oneself but help from the collective to lift the curtains of confusion and competition.

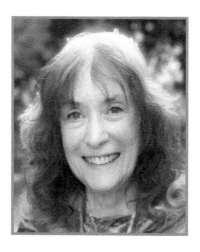

• • ● • •

Nischala Joy Devi was originally trained in Western medicine and is resourced from nearly two decades' experience as a monk. She began to blend Western medicine with yoga and offered her expertise in developing the yoga portion of the Dean Ornish Program for Reversing Heart Disease and co-founded the award-winning Commonweal Cancer Help Program. With her knowledge of yoga and her experience in assisting those with life-threatening diseases, she created Yoga of the Heart, a training and certification program for yoga teachers and health professionals. Nischala was one of the founders of the International Association of Yoga Therapists (IAYT), and serves on the advisory board.

Publications include *The Healing Path of Yoga*, *The Secret Power of Yoga*, *The Secret Power of Yoga* audio book (Nautilus Book Award Winner), *Meditation in the Yoga Tradition* and *The Namaste Effect*.

Nischala Joy Devi

I was a monk for 18 years. My path started with my own seeking. I had no interest in becoming a teacher. I never thought about anything like that, but I had this incredible burning within me to learn the truth, and to learn who I was.

I think the first thing I would say to someone is respect the practice that you've chosen. Have real respect for it, as if it is something that's going to lead you into the light, which it does, into love.

I think that from that, well, like the way the Sufis say, take from the overflow, not from the depth; I think that's what started to happen—this overflow started to come. Then from there, back to your original question, is why I decided to start teaching. Because the fullness was just coming out of me, and it wasn't like I was organizing a class; the class organized me, and people started coming, and saying, "We want to learn."

The difference between a spiritual teacher and a teacher, and this is what I keep saying even in the yoga therapy world, is that you have to keep the yoga in yoga therapy. If you don't keep the yoga in it, it's just Western medicine. For me, the most important thing is the transmission from the teacher to the student, and the student might then become the teacher, and transmit that. Yoga has always been like that. All this that we're doing online now is really difficult for some of us. I just wrote up a whole little etiquette for online, because people are lying down, they're eating, and they pretend it's not like it's a real classroom. I said, "The way I teach is from your feedback, and if I can't see your face, it's very difficult for me to do that." This is why I'm really glad we're doing this as a video, because that's how I've learned to teach, and that's my way of teaching, the imparting of the energy, not just the imparting of the knowledge. Otherwise, it's very interesting because one of the analogies I talk about is the worst punishment that you can give anyone in our society is to put them in solitary confinement. Yet monks crave it. So what's the difference? What is a calm mind, and what is a tumultuous mind? Because that's what happens: you're alone with yourself. Again, I just got an email from one of my friends, and she said, "I found out through this whole isolation time that I actually like myself." I thought, "Yeah, that's a great thing to find out!"

I was originally trained in Western medicine, and I was a physician's assistant.

I come from that, and then I became very disillusioned with Western medicine, very disillusioned with it, and decided to leave it. As I was doing that, I found that there was this emptiness, if you can call it that, that I felt in my heart, that I needed to find out what it was, not necessarily fill it, but find out what it was. What was it yearning for? Serendipitously, I met a man—not a romantic situation, but just a man who then showed me the way to the yoga. As soon as I walked in, I felt that I was home, and I knew why I was there, and then from there started to take classes, and started to learn what yoga really was, not the physical, not the superficial, but that place that was empty in me.

Things weren't seen yet and hadn't come to fruition, and that's why I didn't understand what they were, because I tried to understand it with the mind. The mind can't understand things like that. The heart can. This was not part of my culture. It certainly wasn't part of the medical institution that I was working in. I didn't know where to go. It was one of those things that you don't know what it is, so you can't find the remedy for it.

The first time I saw the picture of Swami Satchitananda, I said to myself, "I don't know what he has, but whatever he has, I want it, and I'm going to do everything I can to get it." Because I saw a sense of peacefulness, but not just peaceful; and there was a sense of joy, underlining that peace. I think that's really, to me, the crux of what's happening in the spiritual world. People are getting it; they may be getting something, but it's not necessarily the depth of joy that allows us, in times like this, in times of need, in times of crisis, to go to that place and find solace.

Because I know, for me, if I'm rushed and I walked into a class, and I don't remember who I am, it's clumsy. Then I have to say, "Okay, I need a minute or so, let me go in," and I do that. I think that the mystical and the practical have to go hand in glove. I think it's not really a bridge that I come back and forth on; it's something that happens when I'm sitting in front of someone. I'm not thinking of the techniques that I want to use, I'm feeling them, and then afterwards, the techniques come in. That's just the way that I function, and I think part of it is after 18 years of being trained like that, and in certain practices, that you don't leave it. I was watching someone practicing a dance step, and they said, "Oh finally, it went to muscle memory." They didn't have to think about it. I think it's like that with the practices. After a while, you're not saying, "Oh, I should be kind to this person, or I should pick up that piece of paper that's on the street." It's not something you think of, it's something you just do.

I think so many people start with a physical practice, because a lot of people feel the physical. I always encourage people, if you pick a physical practice, always pick a subtle practice to go with it, to wrap around the physical. The physical is making your body strong, making your nervous system strong. But then make sure that there's something subtle that you're practicing every day, because then you get the inner, and the outer can meet that. Otherwise, you're just doing the physical, and there's no coordination with the subtle. We have to start feeling with our hearts, as well as our bodies, and our minds. I think most people don't, for various reasons; it's too painful, that's not their way, or whatever. But I think that's what begins to happen.

This one man was sitting there. He actually was a retired physician and he was listening to me. His eyebrows were crossed, he was listening to me, trying to figure all this out. And then he just went like this, and raised one finger. I said to him, "Yes?" He said to me, "I never heard about this Ahimsa stuff before. I didn't know what you were talking about, but then I started thinking about it, and going over my life in the last year, when I've changed this diet. Do you think that's why butterflies land on me now?"

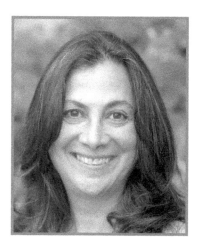

• • ● • •

Lori Bashour co-founded Phoenix Rising Yoga Therapy (PRYT) with her husband, Michael Lee, in 1986 and has been instrumental in its growth and development for over 35 years. Lori has had her own practice as a massage therapist, yoga teacher and adjunct course director.

She now happily settles into her role as Executive Director of PRYT.

Lori Bashour

So one day, I had dusted in Mataji's room, doing all this great cleaning, and then I dusted in Bapaji's meditation chamber, and then I was walking through the woods. And as I was walking through the woods, I went into molecules and my body no longer existed, and I was just, like, that Monet painting where it's all the little dots. I became all the little dots and part of the woods and I wasn't there anymore. I was just breathing.

I create structures for things to grow in, in a way. It could seem, like, because I'm willing to step in the unknown, it just could seem like there's no plan. So there isn't a plan, because I want the plan to be open to grow. I don't want to close it in, like, someone says, you know, "God has more in store for you than you have in store for yourself, so trust God not yourself." I really live by that.

There's "nowhere to go, nothing to do" and I just landed. And for the first time in my life I had a massage. I think I was 25. So that was my first massage and massage wasn't really out then. And it was an amazing experience. And just getting in... It was the first time I was not using my body as a tool and I was being in my body. And it was the first time I was hearing the words of being in this moment, being present—there's nowhere to go or nothing to do. Going on walks in the woods and everything about my life just surrendered into it.

I found that this was a place that I wanted to live. Like the place inside of me was a place I wanted to live. And because everyone at Kripalu was living it that way, I was attracted to staying and so I did. It wasn't the spiritual aspect of the yoga yet; it was waking up in the morning and you just do your yoga and then there's breakfast and then you just do your work and then there's lunch and then you just do your work and then there's dinner. And then you go take a shower and you come back and you get to dance in these white robes and sing and listen to the guru talk. It was a blissful existence. But what was really happening was a cleansing. And really what was happening was that everything underneath was getting triggered.

So I had these things that I had to look at about myself, and have them reflect back to me.

And I found that this was a place that I wanted to live. Like the place inside of me was a place I wanted to live.

Somewhere in that time, something touched inside of me. I think it was before I actually moved in. Something touched me that said, "I want to do this work for the rest of my life." I just want to be here for the rest of life, and this is what I'm going to do. And so I never went back to my apartment in New York. I moved everything out, then came back and moved in.

That was my wake-up moment. It's not when Phoenix Rising started, but when I woke up.

I even got kicked out of the ashram, and that's another story.

But I surrendered to myself. And I realized I received the power of letting go and surrendering and trusting the will of the universe and the will of my spirit. And that the strength was in following my intuition. If I'm led somewhere, I recognize I'm being led somewhere and I'm just going to go there wholeheartedly. All in.

So I went to Sumneytown, and I worked in Amrit Desai's house, cooking meals for the family. And it was at the time when Amrit's son was getting married. So I was behind the veil at the ashram for about a month, but it seemed like a lifetime. I loved every second of it. I was in Mataji's bedroom. She had all these spiritual things and my job was cleaning and dusting everything as well as the cooking in the kitchen. And, you know, Amrit's daughter is there, eating ice cream, and being sassy, being a teenager. She wasn't getting married, her brother was. She was in high school. There was this wedding going on and all the relatives.

My job was also to clean where Swami Kripalu, whom we know as Bapuji, had come and meditated.

What it was called then was selfless service, which I had never done before. You wake up and you do your service. And it was an honor to be serving in the guru's home, and to be there intimately with what was happening. The conditions of all of the people around me. It was a true community in Sumneytown. We had our gatherings; it was intimate. And there was this wonderful thing of somebody going to the store to buy the food, and somebody cooking it. Living in community in a way that can't be recreated in a family.

Even a few weeks ago (this was May 2020), Amrit came up here and we had a healing circle with people who lived in the ashram together. We've been out for over 20 years. People are mourning that time still, remembering that sisterhood and that brotherhood. We knew each other. We still know each other. We hadn't seen some for 20 years, but we still deeply know each other. We share a living experience of service together and a collective mission.

I have my fear, but I also have courage and the courage that I have was to follow. I had the courage to follow my path, strengthened by the community that I was living in at the time, and by the prayers and my connection with my inner self, so they both went together. And my inner self and my prayers, my message is from God, or the heavens, or God's will, and I will just follow it.

We're going slowly now because I want it to be grounded in something, now that everyone's on the same playing field. And understanding that what we are creating in Phoenix Rising is actually an ecosystem. It's not a hierarchy. We're moving from a hierarchy.

So we're moving from that "*me*" into the "*we*" of creating an ecosystem.

And then within that ecosystem are all the people who are stake-holders in Phoenix Rising, and how it's not, like, Michael and Lori are in the center with all these things going out. But it's just more like this ecosystem that's all tied in together and everyone supports and feeds each other. Each entity has a bit of flexibility within it and it moves, and we all play.

So when you change something, you actually lose something. So anytime you change you have to let go because you are losing something. So each stakeholder is going to lose something when we change; we're all going to lose something. How do we address that, and how do we see that what we are gaining is the next phase we are moving into?

And so that's an embodiment practice. That's an embodied knowing that comes from somewhere else, then having an idea and knowing you have to go and find out how to do it. Let's just land together while we close out, so that I can reflect what else might emerge as we distribute this genuine passion into this online virtual world.

I honor a true willingness to try new things, a desire for a legacy that is much more ecocentric than hierarchical. Everyone belonging, everyone having a part, a voice.

A word that's coming to me is "calling." If you have a calling, answer it. If you have a calling, go forth!

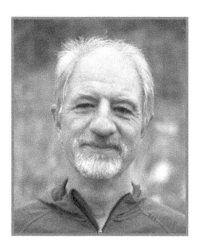

• ● ● ● •

Rob Schware heads the Give Back Yoga Foundation and is President Ex-Officio and Advisor for the Yoga Service Council. In late 2006, Rob brought his two decades of management experience with the World Bank to a second career: helping to grow the yoga service movement. Combining his development and project management expertise in more than 30 countries including India, Indonesia, Turkey, Rwanda and Palestine with his passion for yoga, he formed the organization whose mission is to bring yoga to underserved populations. In 2013, the Give Back Yoga Foundation earned him the International Association of Yoga Therapists' Karma Yoga Award for "extraordinary selfless service in reducing suffering and elevating consciousness through yoga." In 2016, Rob received *Yoga Journal*'s Good Karma award.

He has been married to Alice Trembour for 34 years, which, like yoga, is in and of itself a regular commitment to a practice. They have three children.

Rob Schware

ive Back Yoga Foundation was established in 2007. Again, we really didn't know what we were doing. I think Einstein said, "If we knew what we were doing, it wouldn't be called research." We were sort of piecing this all together, with what we thought were good intentions and a brand name, Give Back Yoga. There was only a pure intention behind it, which is "How may I serve the yoga teachers who have done so much for me in my career at the World Bank; and what talents and skills and knowledge and gifts can I bring to this whole process?"

Well, I'm happy to be here and to be of further service.

The project is a nonprofit called the Give Back Yoga Foundation. I was an official at the World Bank in Washington, DC. I was the lead information technology specialist for 23 years. As part of my health practice as a man, after getting seriously injured as a jogger, quite like many other men, I woke up to the fact that I needed to stretch more.

As I began to practice more, change started happening. It was a greater connection to myself, feeling a greater connection to myself off the mat, feeling I'm connected to a sangha of the yoga studio. These were my friends and we were practicing together, we were studying together.

Then it kind of started expanding, something radiates out in circles of feeling a greater connection to Mother Earth, and then I felt myself waking up and saying, "Oh my God, what is going on—this world is in crisis—drug overdose is the leading cause of death for adults under the age of 50, suicide is the second leading cause of death among veterans, one in three people will get cancer in their lifetime, not to mention our climate crisis?" Gradually, like so many other people, I decided to move from a practice into yoga teacher training.

I started training with Beryl Bender Birch. At the time, and I'll never forget, she would ask questions like "Why do you want to practice yoga? Why do you want to do this work? Why do you want to get started on this path? Because this path is going to lead you to becoming a spiritual revolutionary, and that's not an easy road to follow or something to take for granted, because your life is going to change, because yoga is about service." In a nutshell.

That's how my journey in all of this began.

I think my initiation came, Allie, when I woke up one Sunday morning... I was nearing the end of a 300-hour Ashtanga teacher training program, and I had a "eureka" moment. I said to my wife, "I am simply not going to be a good yoga teacher. There's so many younger people who can teach yoga better than me."

I wanted to work with corporate executives, a milieu I was familiar with for many years. I recall struggling that whole Sunday with questions like "What are my gifts? What's my calling? What can I be doing in the yoga space?" I was in despair. It was fear of failing as a yoga teacher that led me the next morning to get on the phone with my yoga teacher and say, "Beryl, I don't feel I can be a good yoga teacher." I decided instead to start a nonprofit called the Give Back Yoga Foundation. We didn't have any fear of doing that, because we didn't know what we were doing.

I had managed large projects for two decades. I developed pretty solid networking skills and learned team building and how to delegate. Here were yoga teachers wanting to serve their local communities, but not necessarily the best at managing that kind of project as a business that could expand and scale. That was the beginning of my yoga service story.

We shared both the passion for spreading the transformative gift of yoga, as well as the knowledge that yoga and service are intrinsically intertwined. Yoga is/as service. Yoga makes change—it's that simple.

It took me several years to come to an understanding and acceptance of myself as a "manifester" in the yoga industry.

There's an awakening, there's some personal transformation that what was happening in the past for me just isn't working anymore, and I need to change that. At some point, "Oh, wow, look at that, I would just love to share it with my sister and brother and uncle and the people down in the local shelter."

Once I got "cool" with letting go of any attachment to results, everything else seemed to flow like a river.

That combined with some fortuitous things that happened. Our second project request was to support the Prison Yoga Project, founded by James Fox, who has been teaching yoga, violence prevention and emotional literacy at San Quentin State Prison since 2012. His book *Yoga: A Path for Healing and Recovery*, which Give Back Yoga funded, has now been sent free of charge to over 30,000 prisoners. The practices are designed to improve mental and physical wellbeing, which can directly lower healthcare costs among the incarcerated. Prisoners mostly hear about this book by word of mouth, and then request a copy. Prison Yoga Project has trained over 2500 prison yoga teachers in 25 states and seven countries.

This support led to Give Back Yoga's decision to serve as a fiscal sponsor to yoga teachers with "a fire in their belly" who wanted to expand their work and protocol without having to run a nonprofit. We started handling all the tax accounting and some marketing assistance to help scale and elevate the yoga being offered to unserved populations.

All of these programs are led by amazing yoga teachers, each with a fire in their belly. Visionaries who have been working "in the trenches."

I think when you have that yogic experience and feel the deeper connection to yourself, to your brothers and sisters and to our Mother

Earth, you wake up and want to be of service to others. I know this practice works. All I can do is share it with others without attachment towards outcomes. That needs to be the heart of the effort.

Becoming more connected to yourself and, for me, realizing my dharma was to be of yoga service. As soon as I got into that river and that mental state, I felt a greater connection to what I call Supreme Intelligence. Supreme Intelligence was allowing me to commit to a daily yoga and meditation practice and to offer this up to others.

Which then led me to experience just deeper and greater layers of connection and responsibility for everything around me...how I speak and act with my beloved wife, my three children, my friends, and how I treat the Mother Earth. What kind of role and responsibility do I have to my brothers and sisters, to Earth?

It's an uncovering process. What I've discovered in my career in yoga service, Allie, is that yoga and mindfulness are a kind of power plant that can transform collective suffering. A Christian precept says it well: "It is in giving that you receive." I've interviewed for the Give Back Yoga Foundation's blog site and the Huffington Post over 100 yoga teachers who are doing amazing service work in their communities throughout the world. The one theme that is continuous through those interviews runs something like "Working in the jail, working in the shelter, teaching in the treatment center is the best hour and a half of my week"... It's being of service to others.

I've encountered so many professionals who have long-standing careers in accounting, marketing, finance and law who practice yoga and mindfulness. Some of them wake up like I did and ask themselves, "How can I use my skills, knowledge and talents to support the grow-ing community of yoga activists who have dedicated themselves to take their yoga off the mat into their communities, and to work with marginalized and vulnerable communities?"

I think every moment is a choice. I will look back with gratitude for another story about the Give Back Yoga Foundation, which is not my particular story. It's a story that highlights the vital contributions of the dozens of board and advisory members, program directors, staff, yoga teachers, yoga therapists, yoga practitioners, behavioral health specialists, donors, sponsors and yoga practitioners who collectively have made Give Back Yoga what it is today. That story is much larger!

To me, yoga begins when you leave the mat and you begin to know what to do when you are not practicing on the mat. For me, it was realizing my individual dharma as well as our collective dharma as well. I believe our collective dharma has a path and a purpose just as much as any individual path.

I think that is what is clearly being presented to us right now in this time of the climate and COVID-19 crises.

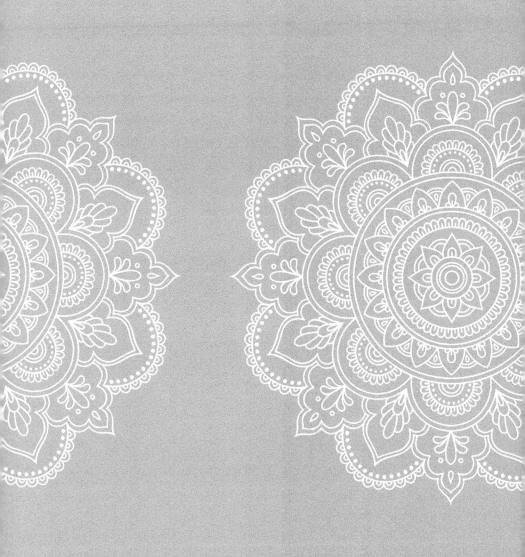

VIII

A New Day After
a Long Night

*Landing in wellbeing and
dreaming the world into being.*

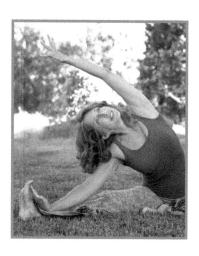

• • ● • •

Monique Lonner is the Director and creator of Soul of Yoga's 300-hour advanced yoga teacher training and IAYT (International Association of Yoga Therapists)-accredited yoga therapy training programs. She has been studying and teaching therapeutic yoga for 20 years. Her specialty is teaching anatomy and physiology to yoga professionals while weaving together science, philosophy and spiritual wisdom. She credits her understanding of yoga and life to the many present-day wisdom keepers who have been her teachers; each offering most profound influences on her current approach to asana and pranayama.

Monique Lonner

As long as I can continue to come back to "How do I know the difference"—well, I know the difference because I know me, and I know my relation to the universe. If I can really sense into that relationship, then it all becomes very clear.

I see that as if there's a keystone moment in my life, and why it's important to do what I do, even when I'm exhausted and want to leave, it's this: it's that I think that yoga therapy is going to help people cross this bridge into a new way of being healthy. And that new way of being healthy is also about being more open in our hearts and minds toward everybody else and understanding, which is the key piece of yoga, that we're all connected. We're connected to each other and we are connected to the earth and you can't help but know that once you start practicing yoga. That's no little thing.

When was I aware that something larger was happening? Probably not until really recently, which is sort of funny. If I look at my path, I started spending so much money on yoga classes that when the studio held teacher training, I thought, well, I'll be a teacher and then I won't have to pay for yoga classes. I became a teacher and then ended up at a yoga retreat and met my husband, Steve. I met him through yoga and ended up in California through yoga and found Soul of Yoga, because I was looking for a job.

That took me down a whole other path of yoga as a spiritual journey. It was just one thing after the next. I take this spiritual aspect of yoga and marry it to the more scientific aspects of yoga that I had been studying in New York, where I'm from. My first teachers had a very anatomical, physiological approach, which is frankly very profound on a certain level. We have facts now how yoga practice impacts this body, the manomaya kosha. Then when I found these facts on the other koshas, it blew me away, so I started thinking, well, everyone should have this experience of both things. It was all just very logical, and then at some point after eight training sessions, I kind of sat back and I thought, wow! Wow! Look at where the universe took me from one place where I was unhappy. And on the ocean of yoga moved me to a place where I'm joyfully happy, but also able to contribute to so many people's lives, which was not my initial intention.

Training teachers to really have both aspects of yoga, to learn how it can help us spiritually, physically, mentally and in training teachers and now, yoga therapists, it is a delight to see them work with people to their full extent. As you were saying, this idea of a star, how it radiates outward and outward, and how that is similar to what is happening now, teachers that we train go and train other teachers and help more people. When I think of it like that, it's almost more than my little mind can hold, the extent that this can reach.

I'm always surprised at the way a training program goes, that it is absolutely, deliciously perfect. Everyone who showed up was exactly who needed to show up. The people who canceled last minute, needed to cancel at the last minute in order to create that perfect incubator of personalities that aren't just sitting there learning but who are inter-acting and supporting each other's growth, so that we all rise together. To me, there's a process that goes behind it, yes, yes. You have to fill out the boxes and the forms and make sure they meet the accreditation standards and you would get the payment schedules done and all of that happens. You build your website, you have your handouts, but that's not what drives me.

What drives me is simply an idea comes and something in me—there's no question that is the right thing to do. I don't question at all.

I have a real enthusiasm around doing some things. When I feel it, I think it's Rumi who says, "It's something that moves in your soul." When people sense that in you, and you're talking to them about something, they sense it, they want to be a part of it. They also know it's right. Because we're seeing each other on another level, besides verbally. That people understand, "Oh yeah, I feel what you're saying. I get it, it's right. It's time for this. I want to do that, absolutely."

If there's a challenge that I face, some people say, "Well, that won't work, that will never work. People aren't going to want to come or that's not financially sustainable"—all the many things that people say. If you have something that is a thought for you and it feels so strong, and there's not even a question in your mind, then you know it's right. Who are other people to tell you that something that hasn't been done before can't work?

Because I can tend to bulldoze other people that way, the universe is the thing that often stops me. I practice that sense of trusting surrender and trusting the natural flow of things just as much as trusting my own ability to get something done. It is really powerful for me. How do I know the difference? Where is the wisdom to know the difference? It's in the svadhyaya. It's in the self-study. If I get really busy and I forget to do my practice, I lose touch with that and then I start pushing where I should surrender or giving up where I should move forward, and the whole balance gets thrown out.

Other people's voices do not represent the voice of the universe. I think that's also the answer to your previous question that if you're so sure, you just felt this, it's so true for you that you need to go do this. Every time you sit down to meditate, or if every time you practice, that comes through so strongly. Don't listen to other people's voices as strongly as you would listen to that voice of the universe, because that's the real one and that comes through the process. It's guided, it's inherent in all of us, we all have that inner connection. The inner Zoom call, I might say, to the higher power. That really is what I try to live by.

We hear that all the time in self-care that awareness is this cure for everybody. And in a very real way, that is true. We see this now in the world, right? If we take care of ourselves and we stay healthy, we have a much greater chance of remaining healthy. When we're not ill, we have less of a chance of making other people ill. I'm sort of taking it from a little bit different standpoint, but our health matters to other people's health. The planet's health matters to our health and our health matters to the planet. So if I'm doing what's healthy for me, which is eating sustainable, organic food, that's automatically better for the planet.

I don't know if I see a separation between what is right for me, truly at that soul level, and what is right for the world.

What is becoming clear to me now, as a leadership perspective, is that health is, as we know, as yogis, that health is not being symptom-free. Health is not "I have this issue, I take a pill, now I'm healthy." Health is a balance of all the koshas. Having a strong body, being strong, and the mind being clear, and the heart being open, and being able to connect to a higher power, if we're going to move through the kosha model.

And I hope, my hope for the world right now is that people will emerge from their fear with a different understanding of what it means to be healthy. That being healthy has so much value on all levels, because it's going to keep us from getting sick. It's sort of a simple concept, but I don't think it's been really widespread, that idea of what real health is. I think that everything has balance. Yoga teaches us that, that nothing can ever really be truly out of balance.

The universe seeks a devotion to life. I think right now that this whole fear of death is really teaching us a devotion to life and yoga is a devotion to life. It's a devotion to being present to everything in one's heart, to following the gifts of your mind. The mind is not an enemy; it's an amazing thing that we can utilize in alignment with the universe—it's a creative force.

To see where we have been using things to define ourselves rather than defining ourselves by the beauty of who we are. I think that, to me, if there were some gift coming in the future that I could be a part of helping people understand, it would be that all of these things that we thought we needed, the cars that we're not even driving right now, all the clothes that we aren't even wearing right now and all of the things that we thought we had to have, don't matter. They really don't. They're fun, but it's not for you. To know who we are. If I can be a part of that, then mission accomplished.

I love pondering this idea of what truly matters. This is a time for many people...I know there are some people who are quite happy in seclusion and they're introverts and they haven't lost their job and they haven't lost a business. There are people who feel pretty good right now. But for all of the people who are struggling, including all the studios, to look at this time and remember, it's hard, but remember that the universe is inherently in balance. There's always day that follows night, night that follows day. Always praying, always birth, always death. That as some things die away, to recognize that the things that we thought define who we were aren't defining who we are because we're still here and they're gone.

What does define us? Who are we? To really use the tools of yoga to feel into who are you without any of those trappings of personality, of ego. We are one, we are one. I hope that that's what gets canonized from all of this difficulty and pain and fear. Because if it's true that every shadow has an equal amount of light, then we've got a whole lot of light coming towards us, eventually.

You'll get just one lens that we use to store the wisdom, in a way that humans can understand it. There are all these other lenses that sort the wisdom into a way that other people can understand it, the

Sufis, the Buddhists, the mystics of all times, and we're all seeing the same thing and we all know that their knowledge is our knowledge and our knowledge is their knowledge, and that we are all one, so I don't see any difference except terminology and labels. I don't know how to say that. I wish there was this beautiful, eloquent statement. It's "we're all one." I think that we know that. The more mystical a set of lenses becomes or a story becomes, the more we just all go back to that center. Going back to the koshas. We all know that the center of joy comes from being together, the real part of us, as you said, the part that matters.

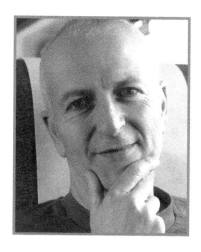

• • ● • •

Leigh Blashki, senior registered teacher with Yoga Australia and Meditation Australia, Certified iRest Teacher and iRest mentor and supervisor, is on the Board of Directors of the International Association of Yoga Therapists (IAYT) and is the Associate Director of iRest Australasia. Leigh was a founding member of Yoga Australia and the founder of the Australian Institute of Yoga Therapy, and served for nine years on several IAYT committees.

Leigh received a Presidential Award at the IAYT Symposium on Yoga Therapy and Research in 2013 and a Yoga Therapy Seva Award in 2017. He regularly presents at international conferences and contributes to journals and books on yoga and yoga therapy.

Over and above his "luminous" teachers, Leigh regards every student, trainee and mentee as a profound teacher who has helped him grow.

As part of his movement into the third phase of life according to the Vedanta tradition (Vanaprastha), Leigh now dedicates more of his time to meditative self-enquiry and mentoring.

Leigh Blashki

True, recognizing that whatever's going on is not something that's been bad. It's not an attack. It's just that this is happening within this broader context of being-ness, if you can call it that. Just existence itself. That a limited part of myself wants to fight against it. And then when I stop the fighting, get out of the way, a perspective comes and this can be just another set of symptoms. And yes, I can acknowledge there is some anxiety and fear, asking, "What does this mean?" And see all the existential stuff and the mortality and those sorts of things, like, of course I'm supposed to be human again.

At times, I felt I was able to still maintain that sense of being-ness that I hadn't had previously with him. It was just remarkable to observe what had changed.

I like that you put it in the present rather than what happened 50 something years ago when I started. I guess it's a continuing and probably a revolving iteration of the understanding of the unqualified non-dual teachings. Most notably, Kashmir Shaivism where there's a greater real feeling of these principles of non-separation and wholeness. Even as we're talking, I would say across time, well, what does that really mean? I mean, I spend hours a week on Zoom with people in the United States and other places. And it's meaningless, these time differences.

I was actually applying these principles of therapeutic relationship, and it's quite about just unconditional positive regard. And all those things I didn't know about all that stuff, but it was happening. It was just unfolding. And so now in the present moment, as I feel into that, it makes sense now for some reason. It comes back to that question of the initiation aspect of it. I don't know how it actually is all initiated, but something is.

And so I guess it was the dance, the unfathomable mystery that we might call that "something else," that "other" which is here in the room; we're calling it in now, not the other way around. And, of course, Kashmir Shaivism speaks to this a lot. Of course, other than that wonderful combination of these primordial energies and the many ways the ancient wisdom traditions represent them.

And now I'm thinking, well, wow, I'm starting to understand by way of feeling what was just unfolding. So this is brand-new mentation that I was actually trusting unconsciously a lot more over the years, natural unfolding in the natural teaching, the natural whatever the god force is, or universal consciousness in other words. That was actually guiding all of this from the word go. And occasionally I accepted that.

Now, to try to make it practical, let's just say for the younger reader, let me see. So, in the teaching process, what I feel is really important, I'll start from the teaching process is being deeply present to allow the resonance to occur. So that by momentarily, to the best of my abilities, which is, of course, always this, just simply being.

It's been a gradual educational process for me of getting out of the way. And again, learning this move from the "*me*" to the "*we*." Getting the "*me*" out of the way so that I can attune to that greater "*we*" field, if you like. And this is, to me, the epitome of self-study. To me, this is an attunement.

So in terms of the yoga therapy students, obviously we discussed it at the time, it wasn't just discussing, we sat quietly before we discussed it. And I just said to them to the effect of, I think I used the word "holy space" or "sacred space," and I just said, "Look, so-and-so is gone, can we just sit and hold him together?" And whether that holding him together was part of his progress or not, they got it. I mean, people who have studied yoga therapy in our training program have had many, many years of yoga practice so they're experienced practitioners.

Let's look at the relationship side of it. And can we keep remembering this is about co-creating better relationships.

My yoga journey started because of health crises. My body is like a 1950 Chevy pickup truck with rusting everything, yet what a work horse it is that I've been carried in.

But the perspective comes in saying, well, "If that's what it is, am I going to go backwards and fight against it and lock down, or do I just keep open?" It hasn't been easy. It's been really hard; I have to say, it's been a real challenge. It's been a focus of my personal practice, I guess the last three years, to say, "Welcome this in, welcome this in. What have you to say? Well, come on in." Kind of like walking into the unknown. Welcome it all in.

So welcoming, I guess, is the key feature at the moment. Do I have a preference not to be there? Sure. Welcoming the presence, at least welcome what is because it is here, and it might well be the next step, the next messenger.

If I think way, way back, my first recorded experience of these traumas is at the age of six when I was in hospital for my first open heart surgery. I was the fourth person in Australia to have open heart surgery, at the age of six, and I don't recall trauma at that time. I just recall things went on and there were horrible events, injections and being in an oxygen tent and three weeks in the hospital as a kid; I felt like I was being dumped there.

But being taken home, literally being carried across the main road from the hospital into a car by my father, is a very, very powerful image. And with that was a sense of there was something whole here. There is something caring behind all of this that can be trusted. It presented in the form of a father at that time. But in later years, I scroll down a little bit in my own thinking and cadence of therapy. Really, what was that? Was it my father, or was that a greater sense of trust and faith that is innate? Even that the mind is saying, "I am afraid. What's going to happen?" And innate trust, yet I guess all that has enabled me to bring that trust further into the therapeutic relationship and teaching and vice versa. They support each other. We know that this thing's always two ways, there's no one-way street.

So it's my daily on-the-mat practice, it is my dedication to releasing the mental tensions through some form of psycho-emotional practice. And commitment every day to connection with, I'll just use the word "Nature." But you understand what I mean by that is something more than just this. It is a lovely garden. It's like the deepest component of all of that. That's because as I talk, I can't talk properly unless I connect with Nature. It's all around me and I'm looking at it.

So you look at these trees and loving the bushes and other things every so often, because that helps me to ensure that I'm connecting with you. You see that whole sense, you're not just going into the head space; I can show the wholeness of Nature. And I think of yoga in the traditional sense; it's a very Nature-based practice. You go right back to its roots.

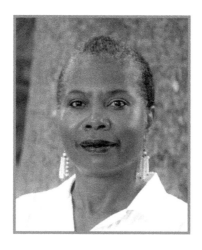

• • ● • •

Jana Long is the executive director of the Black Yoga Teachers Alliance (BYTA) and Power of One Yoga, based in Baltimore, Maryland. She is a yoga therapist, Ayurvedic lifestyle consultant, meditation facilitator and mentor who specializes in the therapeutic application of yoga to inspire and empower people 60 years and older to revitalize their bodies and spirits with practices focused on the full spectrum of aging and wellness. Jana has traveled globally to study meditation and contemplative practice with a diverse yoga and spiritual community. She has extensive experience in media, non-profit and for-profit management, and is responsible for the visionary leadership to guide BYTA through its growth and development.

Jana Long

It's not that linear for me. I try to be open and sometimes either it's an arousal, it could be a momentary thought, it could be in a dream. I don't know where it comes from. It just comes and I am the kind of person who doesn't try to think things through to the finish. If something arises within me that requires me to take action, I take action just to see where it will go, if it's what I should do. Because time will tell, or the evolution of it will tell. And as a result, I've had many different experiences. It's just like that feeling in that church as a little girl: something just wells up in you and you just go for it and see where it goes, see where that road goes. You can't be afraid to go down that road.

But that's our opportunity to look at what we create. To create with intention and consciousness not unconsciousness. And until we do that moving from "*me*" to "*we*," that's going to be a big part of it. How we create and what we create. It's so incumbent on each of us to look within ourselves. What am I consciously creating because I'm bringing that forth into the world?

But the interesting thing was, as a child, I felt that I could feel that thing, whatever it was that moved them to get up and dance in ways that you could not consciously dance. You just totally let yourself, you released yourself to this feeling. I remember that and would do my little dancing and all as a child. And I wasn't a very shy child. I remember once walking up the aisle of the church and just belting out this song, "Yes, Jesus loves me!" But I'm three. I'm three years old, and I could feel something moving in that experience of being in that church.

They said they "got the Holy Ghost." That's what they called it.

But with my grandmother, we traveled South, back home. Another experience again going South; now I'm older, I'm eight years old and this time in Georgia with a great-uncle, same thing, two churches on the block. And I mean these are black communities, outhouses, no indoor plumbing, lots of fresh food, however. And also, my experience with the earth because everyone's farming. It's an agricultural community and food is exchanged and yet I never saw it as a poverty experience because of the love in the home and the deep learning to appreciate the earth.

I was side by side with my grandmother: planting, harvesting, canning, swapping food with neighbors and everything.

I wasn't so much seeking. I guess initially I was seeking religion, but I could never land in any of them comfortably. So I turned to astrology when I had the capacity on my own. Wanting to understand, I began to seek. First there was astrology, then in high school a classmate turned me on to Buddhism and chanting.

The first book I bought was by J. Krishnamurti. It's called *The First and Last Freedom*. Now I'm in my late teens and trying to understand what is the nature of self and who am I, what am I? I would say astrology became the foundation for a study of, or an understanding of Ayurveda's meaning and how the understanding of the energetic qualities are part of our known universe. How it is me and how it is everything around me. The qualities and energies of masculine and feminine that are beyond an embodiment of gender in people, as primary qualities of energy, of creation. All I can say is one thing unfolded into the other.

Yoga came along quite accidentally. In our gym classes at school, there was a posture I always loved doing. In school, they called it the bicycle, but what it essentially was, was shoulder stand. And then move into the halasana, or plough pose. I just love doing that on my own. I had no idea that was connected to anything called yoga, but it was something that I did on my own. One day I happened to be scrolling through TV stations and there was Lilias Folan on TV back in the early 1970s. And just in that moment there she was coming up on to her shoulders there. And it was like, "Oh, hey, there's that thing I like to do." So there was this plate of yoga and I began to watch her program for the physical practices. I was already pretty well steeped in searching and devouring many books.

I didn't have very many friends I could discuss these things with, without them thinking I was some kind of weirdo, which was the label that I lived with for quite a long time. "Oh, you know Jana, she's all into that weird stuff."

And so I learned to hold that part of myself sacred for me and only reveal it to people I knew that I could have a conversation with. Then I met other people from different countries who were more open, and we would sit in and have fun and basically just discuss these things. That was the beginning of it all. That's how it all began.

And so I was just curious about people who understand how we live in different ways. I felt what I was getting from what I was reading was not so dogmatic. If it works for you, that's fine. Choose what serves your life, but that does not mean that people who do not ascribe to that are wrong. It's interesting to hear how they perceive and see the world.

I didn't come out of the shell until the late 1990s. It was a good 30 years again, because of largely learning that I don't go along to get along, that's not been my path...to go along to get along. I've always walked my own path in many ways. Maybe alongside and in step with the crowd sometimes, but I'm not in the crowd, I'm offside from the crowd. In most of the cases, I want to go off in a different direction. Then I was in my late 40s.

The first thing that I think helped to cultivate serious practice was a time, again in my quest for religion, where I practiced Islam for a while, which is a very disciplined religion. You're making prayer five times a day; you've got to stop what you're doing to do that and make that a habit. The fasting month is an incredible honer of discipline. And getting into fasting for Ramadan helped me to really see with that citta within myself, how that works and which of those different arousals of my nature can I practice the brahmaviharas with? Can I restrain myself from the most basic of our instincts? And to do that year after year.

Until I found that there were just other aspects of Islam that didn't work for me, but there were certain wonderful rituals in it. Those were some of the early practices that came into my life that helped me to understand how to establish a practice, a consistent practice.

Just go down, take a step, start walking down the road. And either you'll get to a new destination where you have to turn or turn around and come back, or go in a new direction. Just go. As Nike says, "Just do it," and trust what arises within you. Where else is it going to come from? I don't do things that other people think are good for me to do unless I feel...I have to feel it germinate within me, not because somebody said it's good for you or you should do this. Whenever I've done that, it hasn't worked out very well. I started to trust my own vision for my life and to move with it and not be afraid. Just go.

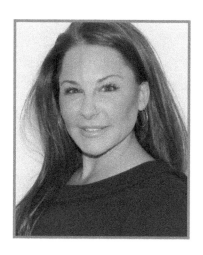

• • ● • •

Heather Mason is the founder of The Minded Institute, a yoga therapy training organization focusing on mental health and empowering yoga and health professionals to integrate yoga therapy into healthcare. She spent three years developing and transforming her mind and sharing her yoga teaching with nuns in Buddhist monasteries in South East Asia. She has trained and been guest faculty at the Boston Trauma Center, Boston University School of Medicine, Maryland University of Integrated Health and Harvard Medical School Mind–Body Medicine, before moving to the UK.

Heather is the Secretariat of the All-Party Parliamentary Group on Yoga in Society and works with the UK House of Commons to coordinate and establish initiatives through parliamentary procedures in the UK government. She founded the Yoga in Health Care Alliance (YIHA), which she runs with other directors. YIHA now trains yoga professionals throughout the UK. In 2020, Heather co-founded Healthflix, an initiative where world leaders in mind–body science and techniques offered free talks and skills to the public during the pandemic. When she isn't working, Heather is dancing, writing music and playing with her magical little dog, Minnie Monkey!

Heather Mason

Maybe that's the piece coming from my spiritual practice, that my teacher told me that if you hold an opinion, and you attach to an opinion, you're at the lowest level of mind. So you always have to know that what you perceive and think is subject to being incorrect, inaccurate, and should be able to be reformed. And I really reform, rather than perform. I think that that really serves me, because if someone gives me new information, and my mind goes, "Okay, here's a new way of saying the whole thing," it does it very quickly. And that's because of my practice.

It's not a story I often tell, but I actually was on an anti-malarial [drug] while in Costa Rica by myself at the age of 18. And I had almost a psychotic break off of the back of it. Reality unfolded for me in a way that was so profound, but I didn't have the foundation to manage. And I came back to New York, and I wanted to be admitted into a psychiatric hospital, actually. And this very wise psychiatrist who I didn't want to go back to, because I wanted to be fixed, said, "Unfortunately, you're describing a very special experience. And although your anxiety is crippling you, you're not psychotic, you're describing very profound things. And all I can do is give you something to manage your anxiety."

I was furious. That sent me to so many different quarters of the world, actually. But the very first one was Gurumayi in New York. I had no expectation of who she was, or what I was meant to do there, but I was just given a private audience without even asking. So this felt very much like it was karmic for me. And I thought she was going to say, "Okay, child, I fix you now."

She didn't. She said, "You must go to India and seek the next stage in your path. Here's a mala practice." I didn't know what to do with it. I didn't understand. And that was it.

That's when my message really started to move through yoga instead, because I realized through breathing and moving, asana and pranayama, that my experience would be more accessible to others, and that the physiological changes would happen more readily.

I sat through that for two years, 16 hours a day, on and off, for two years with that level of suffering. It just gave me something, it gave me the power, I think, to help other people to be able to help their pain, to not be frightened. And to just keep going. "Okay, what do I need to do next? What knowledge am I lacking? How can I make this easier for people than it was for me?"

So then I was lucky enough to be able to create a program at Boston Medical, at the Boston University School of Medicine, an elective. And then that became another stepping stone. And when I came back to the UK, I had that underneath my belt. And then I got invited to speak at Parliament about this, and then somebody else invited me. And then, suddenly, I'm moving in this direction of "Okay, how do we consider this as a society?" Some things I feel like I've worked really, really hard to achieve, and other things have just happened. And I felt like maybe this was meant to be my life path.

I've always tried to understand where people are coming from. I think that's one of the other things that's made it really possible for me in transforming those relationships, I have never ever felt that anything was impossible. I always felt I just needed to understand something different from what I know now. Think outside of the box. And I have not taken my lead as to how to succeed moving forward from anybody else. I've just trusted what's come from my meditation. "Okay, what am I not seeing? How do I view this differently? What does this person need to hear to be willing, for example, to be open to creating the party parliamentary group?" And I also recognize that as somebody on the spiritual path, that nobody can be used for something, like as a stepping stone. Like I need this person for this, so I'm just going to pull them out and work with them in that particular way, manipulate the situation so I can have what I want.

A lot of people that I work with in health policy, they've become my friends. Because that relationship has to be part of the process of growth. And they won't be on board for the long haul otherwise, and my life won't be imbued with any meaning, if everybody's just my colleague. Because I'm working too much, so there has to be a real connection. And I think that that enduring connection also has made a real difference. My commitment is to creating a sangha around my mission.

If there's somebody that can unlock the key, I really listen. And I hear what matters. And I have also an entrepreneurial mind with everything else out there. That's the connection. It's a spiritual kind of entrepreneurial mind. Could we just talk a bit, where's the creation bit here? That's it. That's what matters to you. And that's what matters to me. And I've been listening long enough to actually hear rather than tell you.

I think that that is so incredibly vital. And people do want to talk. If you really want to listen to what they have to say and say what's important to them. They want to talk. And most people, at least the people that I meet, are passionate about something. I'm probably not going to have success with somebody who is totally focused only on themselves.

I don't know what my understanding of it is. It's just an energy. It's not a named thing. It's not that I sit there and say, "Ah, it's here now." It's just, I'll sit there, and there's a very different energy that will come up with ego. Like, I want this, I want this, I want this so much. And that doesn't tend to bear that kind of fruit, as opposed to "Okay, what does the world really need?" It's getting to the crux of that. And all I can describe is, it's like a flow inside myself. It's like when I arrive there, it feels alive. It feels clean, it doesn't feel agitated. And there might be later, a lot of dross and difficulty to make something actually happen. But the idea of the project just seems fluid, clear.

I watch very closely to what people want. I'm always paying attention to that. I'm really trying to understand what people need. I think the first thing is real listening. I really listen to my students in the training, because the Minded Institute is always morphing. And I know that some of my team wouldn't like me to at times, but I'm hearing the students, I'm open. People who criticize you kindly are not trying to chip away. They see something in you, and they want you to grow.

I think one of my leadership skills is being able to take critique as an opportunity. And that has always allowed me to grow.

The next is to understand and look at people's ability to work collaboratively on what my bigger vision is, by understanding what their skill base is. I watch these leaders who are bossy. And I think, oh, they're so much more successful than I am, because they tell people what to do. And people just fall in line. But I could never come to the world in that way. I couldn't sleep with myself at night if I made people feel suppressed.

Maybe it's part of not making me feel how I was growing up, when I couldn't be myself. So it's just that constant willingness to expand. And then alongside that, also knowing—and I'm very bad at this—when expansion is no longer necessary. And when what you planted needs to take root and you just take a moment and you wait, and you also trust. So that you're not constantly, constantly growing and changing and transforming every second. Because you can't keep up with that either.

I think it's very hard to trust. And I think it's hard to have the balance between being a very energetic person, if you want to make change and then letting go. Or if you're somebody who always lets go to realize that you also need to be active in the world. But it's that process, finding how you need to flow, not necessarily based on how many more emails and conversations you need to have, but like, "Okay, this is my edge." It's me telling myself and maybe the universe is speaking it to itself saying, "That's enough now." Sometimes I don't feel like I'm actually...that it happened.

I teach all the time. Do this, do this, do this, this has this benefit, this has this benefit. But that's not how it works for me. I need to sit, and I've done enough meditation to say, "What do I need?" So there isn't this practice. The first practice is the honest awareness of what I need in order to meet the energy and to restore myself. Sometimes it's ujjayi breath, which I do a lot of, at different rates. Sometimes my body and mind say to me, "Just watch us. We can't transform anything more right now. Hold on to this waiting." And I honor that. Sometimes I need to go to Nature. And I need something to reabsorb from. And I know that, too.

So the ultimate first bit is the awareness of what am I truly needing and honoring it. And maybe testing a few things out, and not pushing through at that time. Because that time is not about any pushing through. And then sensing into what needs to happen next, what needs to happen next. Sometimes it's loving kindness for myself and for the world. Sometimes it's weird stuff like going to the forest and basically lying on the ground in a star shape for an hour and doing nothing and looking up at the sky. Sometimes I write music; it's going back to writing music.

But it's that same quality, I guess, that I was talking about. I've never thought about that; it's just listening to myself. It's not telling me that I must do that thing. It's saying, "What do I need to hear, to be aligned?" And then focus on it. It's the same that I do with people, rather than telling them.

There are some sayings in the Buddhist canon that there isn't one panacea. Anybody who thinks that they can just come back to one practice and it will always serve them will be disappointed. And that the true practice is the self-awareness to understand what you need in a moment.

There is light in me and I trust myself. And even if it is hard, and even if I am confused, I believe in that light. And that light never goes out. And as I operate in integrity, the doors of my path continue to flow, opened almost in this magical way.

I don't pretend to be better than who I am. I'm very imperfect and screwed up like the rest of us. I don't want to say that I'm other than that. That's such an important part of this path is saying, "I'm not a guru. I struggle and I'm real. And I'm frightened."

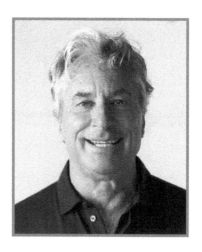

• • ● • •

Lorin Roche was lucky enough to begin practicing asana, pranayama and meditation in 1968, and he still feels like a beginner—every day. He was trained as a meditation teacher in 1969–1970 and has been sharing the delight ever since. Lorin is the author of six books, including *Meditation Made Easy*, *Meditation Secrets for Women* and *The Radiance Sutras*. At the University of California at Irvine, his master's degree work focused on the injuries and developmental crises provoked by meditation and opening the chakras. His PhD research was on the language of inner experience in meditation—the way meditators describe their inner worlds. Lorin is the founder of Instinctive Meditation, grounded in extensive research and experience, teaching an approach designed to match one's individual nature. He serves on the faculty of Esalen Institute, 1440 Multiversity, Kripalu Center for Yoga and Health, Loyola Marymount University and SAND Science and Nonduality. Lorin lives in Marina del Rey, California, with his yogini shaktini wife, Camille Maurine.

Lorin Roche

nd when we meditate, we are actually activating survival genius, adaptive genius. So that's why I say that meditation is instinctive. It's built into every human body and we each have our own way, and it helps people function at their best. Meditation helps you assess the crisis, whatever it is, the challenges, and then find the energy centers in your body, line them up, make a mélange, make a mix, a dance mix just to meet that challenge of using your life energies and your instincts. Match that and save the day.

The essence of it is that yoga in its essence is falling in love with the prana. It's jumping into the dance of prana, and there's a certain duality of "I'm a body–mind system, I am the flow of prana," and then separating a little, and I'm a body of prana that's flowing through me.

Half an hour of meditation in the morning enriches the entire day so incredibly that it's as if I just came back from a year-long fantastic vacation, and yet just half an hour has gone by. And then I can go and function. And everything that I do, I do better after meditation. And then perhaps a meditation time before dinner is a chance to fine-tune again, review the day, learn all the lessons and then start fresh. So that keeps on rocking 52 years later. I still need it.

If we take the language, the original language used to describe yoga and put it in modern English, we could say with these practices are ways of falling in love with the functioning of pranashakti, with the genius of pranashakti, which is dancing everywhere, including in these bodies and in the space between us and all the people that we interact with.

But there's aesthetic rapture also that any fluctuation of pranashakti is genius, and when we behold, we fall in love. And then there are times in that when our entire being is as if suspended. It's hard to talk about it in English, because it implies stillness, but it's not. It's not stillness. It's an immersion in the flow that's so total.

We can take yoga to mean connecting. Literally, it's connecting or joint. The word "yoga" or the word sound "yug" is here in the word joint, conjunction, and the old Greek word for married which is *syzygy*. So the sound, the Y sound in yoga, it's been used in all sorts of contexts, to bringing things together, joining, connecting. And connection is magic, so when we're talking about yoga, we're talking about the magic of connection, the art form of it, the love nature of it, and the science of it, because each of our connections have their own world of magic.

I feel like I awaken to that urge to share again and again every few years, and then I retire. So over the last 52 years I'll be really active for a few years, and on fire with missionary zeal. And it would be the yoga sutra or some book on meditation, or the Radiance Sutras. And the first time was after about a year of practicing yoga and meditation. It was 1969 and I was at the University of California at Irvine, and the whole campus was rioting against the Vietnam War.

And I had already studied the Vietnam War, because I was raised as a warrior. I was raised with guns, hunting, fishing, sailing, skiing and surfing, and diving. That's what a man does.

And I'd been hunting in the afternoon with my father, and I would go out in the morning and shoot wild turkeys and bring them back and feed everybody. So I was raised in this world, raised probably to be a warrior, maybe work for a think tank plotting military strategies. And then I started meditating, and it was like, blam, that's over. This is amazing. After about a year of practicing, I started a club on campus. I would have teachers from Esalen come down to teach every other weekend and give students course credit. The university gave me an office, and so I would be walking in and saying, "Excuse me, excuse me, excuse me," as I'd go through the crowd of people rioting against the Vietnam War, and go to my office, like, "Excuse me. Can I use my phone for a minute?" Call somebody, and then leave, like, "Here, you guys take over my office."

So we were doing meditation and tai chi and body work, Rolfing—I had Rolfers coming to the university and doing sessions. Yoga teachers, dance teachers, art therapists, Rolfing, tai chi, and Gestalt therapy and Jungian analysis. And this combination, I find, is incredible. It's the yoga tradition, and the tantra yoga tradition, and in using Gestalt therapy and the insights from Jung, and what dance teachers and Rolfers were evolving in terms of somatics, letting that be a way of receiving the genius of the Sanskrit. I found that it's been 52 years now, that integration, that mandala—that's what I had always loved. I find it just worked. It all worked so beautifully.

Yoga can waken up all of our senses so intensely that our ordinary experience has this startling artistic quality. A glass of water, seeing your friend, listening to music. In yoga, the senses are called the indriyas, which means the companions of the divine. The senses are portals to the divine, all of them.

The mystery is that there's no one technique that works for everybody. It's a hunt. It's a challenge. It takes everything you have as practice or as an explorer to jump and find what works. That's the mystery. It's always a challenge.

Our practice has evolved. Lately, the last few months, my meditation has been thrilling and rich, but last year, this is 2020, last year there was about six months where I didn't know what to do in meditation. I would sit over there at four in the morning and go, "What? I don't even recognize myself." But then I'm 70. It could be this happens. "Who is? What is? What? What are the doorways? What? What? Where?" It was months of just darkness and fog.

Now, I think there are people who are so well put together that they don't need to meditate. At least when I meet people, I occasionally meet people who are functioning so beautifully, so I think they have secret practices that they do yet they don't realize they are yoga. But I need classical tantra yoga meditation practices to keep me tuned to function at my best.

As a society, we need people to be functioning at their best. Because actually human beings are good in a crisis. We've been bred over hundreds of thousands of years to be adaptable and to be able to survive almost anything. We're all descended, every single one of us, descended from incredible people who walked barefoot across a thousand miles of snow holding a baby and figuring out how to melt some water and eat along the way. We're all descended from people who found their way through the jungles, who survived volcanoes. So our bodies are tuned to survive and adapt, and meditation is actually an emergent function of the genius of survival that's built into the human body.

The Radiance Sutras are there to remind us that there are 112 doorways into meditation, into ecstatic experience in everyday life, and that there are even more. And each of us, we have our own favorite pathways. Everyone I've ever met already knows one or two of the doorways in the Radiance Sutras, maybe many, and it's a reminder. "Oh, yeah. I know that. I didn't realize that that was my meditation practice. Oh, yeah, I was just thinking about it. Oh, that is my meditation." So it's there to remind us of the richness, that there are a tremendous variety of doorways.

So realize there is something for you. There is a style of meditation for you. Find it. Find that way that thrills you so much that you're glad to be alive and you feel your body–mind system come alive and function best.

The interest in meditation is astounding in the modern West. Just in the United States, there's something like, according to U.S. government statistics, something like 35 million people who now practice meditation. And other studies show that it's on a wish list, it's on the to-do list of another 35 million. So maybe a third of the total population is actively interested in meditation. So it's very important to realize that there are at least 100 different major techniques. It's not about sitting still and trying to blank your mind, which is what everyone is thinking. That's actually a harmful practice for most people. Sitting cross-legged and trying to blank your mind will wreck your knees and your mind.

So it's important to discover what's healthy. There's this tremendous desire among almost everyone to be able to meditate. It's important, and we have to get better as teachers to help people discover their particular way.

You want to approach your meditation practice with playfulness, exploration, kind of like a hobby. You want to make it almost like a vice, an indulgence, something that you're sneaking off to meditate. It's not virtuous. You fall in love with a particular sutra, you learn it by heart, or just go and do the thing that it's talking about. For example, one of the verses is music, and it also means stringed instruments like the guitar or a sitar. So it's a string and also the strings of the heart. So immerse yourself in the rapture of music. You know what you love. Go there. Tend to each note, each chord rising up from silence and dissolving again.

And this word "tend" is a pun on "tantra," which is our word for tender, and "attention" or its cognates, which are cousins to the word "tantra," which means to stretch or extend.

Immerse yourself in the rapture of music. You know what you love. Go there. Tend to each note, each chord, rising up from silence and dissolving again. Vibrating strings draw us into the spacious resonance of the heart. The body becomes light as the sky, and you, one with the great musician, who is even now singing us into existence.

All around you, you can actually see the genius of life functioning. And grab a little moment, and even for two seconds, just breathe with an appreciation of the genius of life. And in this way you'll begin to trust your own instincts and trust the instinctive flow in the people around you.

Passing Through

Not knowing the way
yet fearing not
we sway,
wobbling between and
betwixt it all.
Shall we move and dance
playing with sun and moon?
or sit in trance with stillness askance?
The gate appears and disappears.
Each note, each tone
each taste and
each savory
sensation
pulls and pushes us all
into the emerging dream
of no more words.
And sacred time appears
bowing now
amidst the thunder.
We shall
tell the story
of the space
between the directions
while
running and walking
standing
sitting and lying down.

As the sun steals the night and
the ice feeds the stream
a thunderous roar opens
and the holy flame
keeps us silent, together.

We are passing through the gate
of dawn,
together.

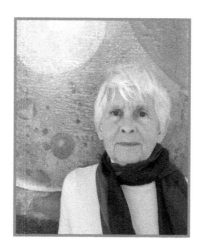

• • ● • •

Amy Kline Gage worked with Dean Ornish, MD, of the Preventive Medicine Research Institute in Sausalito, CA, teaching yoga for coronary artery disease patients for the LifeStyle Heart Trial Research Participants over 40 years. Their work proved that coronary artery disease, and, later, certain types of prostate cancer, can be prevented and reversed. Born into a family of yoga and meditation practitioners, and a devoted spiritual practitioner, Amy studied Anthropology and taught yoga classes with medical applications for more than four decades. She has written about Tibetan psychiatry and the LifeStyle Heart Trial Research Participants. Amy served as the second president of the International Association of Yoga Therapists. She is married, has four daughters, five grandchildren, and a joyful dog, Bella, and lives in Southern California.

Postscript

Dedicated to the memory of Allie's father, Elliott Middleton Jr., MD, an immunologist whose pioneering teaching, and research and writing furthered his field and contributed to the quality of healthy life for people around the world. And to the memory her mother, from the Blackford family who helped introduce a special fish to the markets in New York two centuries ago. May angels sing them to their rest.

COVID-19 and yoga therapy: COVID as a social disease

COVID-19, as a social disease, changed human activity around the world. The infection spreads through the breath and touch. Usually, these two experiences tend to bring people together physically and emotionally and have since we evolved on two feet; but COVID has had other effects, not so gentle. It can kill, changing human contact for closeness and friendship to deadly consequences and debilitating disease, and, for too many, death.

Worse, it has become a political contagion as well as a physical disease. Around the world, distrust has isolated, fragmented and destroyed as this disease gains ground, claiming more lives and disrupting our social interactions from work and school, to family and group gatherings everywhere. Medical supplies to possible vaccines are seen as manipulatable by devolving systems of extreme power and privilege.

Yoga therapy can help heal the planet and contribute to the healing of the COVID scourge on life. A grandiose statement, nonetheless true. We consider cooperation and working together necessary in our work with all conditions and all people. COVID allows us a chance to demonstrate the beauty and efficacy of gentle attention, well-applied service, and successful outcomes.

A powerful tool identified as *hope* is where healing starts within, for so many instances and for so many people. Hope gives energy and revitalizes the mind and body through a positive relationship with others. Cooperation with other healthcare and public health professionals becomes an opportunity to expand our presence and to sense possibility on new horizons. In this world fighting a tiny virus, the one thing we need and crave to co-evolve becomes cooperation, working together to confront this shared threat. It becomes necessary to work in optimism and see the outcome as positive. That comes from faith in life and grounded in transformative process. It makes us more resilient, softer and more effective in working together.

Yoga therapy added to the arsenal of defenses against COVID would round out the already simple requirements of:

1. protect ourselves

2. avoid large gatherings

3. wear a mask for your sake and those around you

4. wash hands frequently and well

5. maintain physical distancing of at least six feet between you and others.

From a yoga therapy perspective, we could add:

1. meditate to keep the mind relaxed and focused

2. breathe as if your life depended on it—fresh, clean air

3. maintain body tone and health with asana practice

4. eat carefully to avoid weight gain and keep healthy

5. be kind whenever possible—it's always possible—to expand your
   faith and spiritual life.

As mentioned in the Dedication, the Shri Vidya Yantra can show us
how to do this. See her, let her in and feel the way your entire being
relaxes and begins to quiet the mind, poise the spirit and connect us
to timeless healing and trust which passes understanding and makes
us see the light. That is the function of practicing with the Shri Vidya
Yantra and other portals of potential; it works through us and among
and between us since time and space immemorial and throughout our
shared human history.

Amy Kline Gage

Appendix 1

The Interview Process

How do we learn to build the capacity to initiate and implement transformative practices in research, community, organizations, larger systems and beyond? The questions that I posed to every single yogi and wisdom-giver form a vital step in the invitation to explore how contemplative inquiry practices sustain integrative leadership development and systems transformation.

These questions follow a blend of techniques. They combine Joseph Campbell's Hero/Heroine's Journey archetype and the Theory U prototyping model (the Theory U prototyping model is an awareness-based change management process researched and developed through the MIT Presencing Institute in Cambridge, Massachusetts, USA).

Starting with a great deal of curiosity bound up with much of what I had discovered as a long-term meditator, yogi and social presencing practitioner, I wanted to learn whether this moving from *"me"* to *"we"* consciousness is reflected in perceptions, actions and behaviors; how does a yoga-based awareness mirror or match a social presencing awareness? The interviews were designed to ground in practice and a certain outlook, a natural conversational framework using deep dialogue practices.

Finally, our collective search will continue further, I suspect, especially as we navigate more fully in the "corona time" evolving on the planet. How does personal transformation set the stage for altruistic innovation practices? How might this lead to greater impact, for the broader social good and connection with all beings?

Co-evolving a "presencing approach"

The interview questions follow a dialogue-inspired listening practice and the distinctive path of the star-shaped prototyping model embedded in the Theory U process. The same pattern runs throughout each interview, with similar progressions, commentaries and narratives bringing new and different insights from yogi to yogini.

We begin with initiation and invocation. What is the origin of somebody's inspiration? What is the spark or vision they see, feel or sense? Then we move on to connection. How does somebody's inspiration move on to be potentially actionable? How might it be that somebody could actually follow through with a process of doing based on their inspiration from the practice of being?

Next, we move on to the clarification of the vision. How does one clarify and refine their vision? What help should one seek, what help or resources does one need? How does someone find the confidence to make new strides, break new ground based on little more than inspiration or guidance from universal life force and ultimate potential?

From here, co-initiation is vital. With a vision in place, with actionable goals underpinning it and the knowledge needed to give it legs to move, how does one establish that core network of people, collaborators, experts and team members that any venture needs in order to succeed? This is often an intimate process as one searches out those who share their deepest cares and concerns, who feel passionate about the project, the vision, and who can help to nurture it into fruition. It's a lot to ask of a team; it's a lot to trust a team when Spirit is guiding the vision.

Crystallization comes next. With all of the above in place, how does one adopt a landing strip, an actual space and place, a context and environment in which it is safe to experiment? Heart and mind follow closely as we dialogue about the experiments; how, in actuality, did each Yoga Radical experiment? What did they actually do? With what, where and with whom? How did they communicate the transformation and what were they learning or trying to learn? What helped to establish and sustain an enduring sense of curiosity and compassion? What fostered the courage to deeply engage in their ideas, to feel safe to fail fast? What can those seeking to learn from them take from their life lessons? What should they avoid that may have delayed or impaired the process of their inspiration taking form at scale?

Then, finally, the outcome emerges. From the initial vision, through the process of building a team, actualizing and realizing the heart's desire while dreaming the future into being, we arrive at the end. What does the fruit of one's search look like? What is the "new" for each of these innovators? What is the thing that they developed and then birthed? What new star has truly landed?

In some of the stories, you will notice a favorite quotation, a saying or sutras from the life lessons shared as foundational sources of inspiration. They are heartening and educational, they are insightful, they are sometimes a little bit intimidating, yet they are all worth taking into consideration as you continue on your path, on your journey.

As a finishing step, you will find a few reflections, some further views from the guidance received from these inspiring and diverse Yoga Radicals. They have cleared our way into the future through their paths of practice. They are willing to pass their inspiration on to you and all others seeking to take their first (or ten thousandth) step.

Shaping Change and Healthy Social Innovation with Theory U and Mindful Dialogue and Embodiment Practices

When I conducted the interviews, I was actually looking at an image of the Theory U prototyping model, with the core aspects reaching out like a five-pointed star. There, in the space in front of me, was my map for each hour-long video dialogue. I needed to remain in a deeply generative state in order to create an opportunity for each interviewee to express from a natural embodied presence, not from anything prepared or from memory. This was a way to activate a resonant relational field during the time that we engaged in dialogue. This practice is part of a very particular path of generative listening, which is illustrated in the image below.

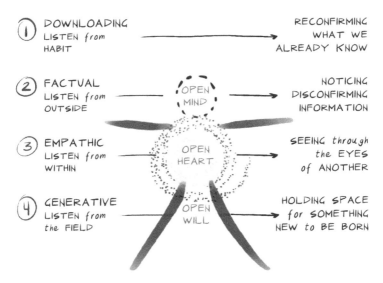

Four Fields of Listening
The Essentials of Theory U—www.ottoscharmer.com

Levels of Listening is a practice from the Presencing Institute (www. presencing.org).

When you operate from Listening 1 (downloading), the conversation reconfirms what you already knew. You reconfirm your habits of thought: "There they go again!" When you operate from Listening 2 (factual listening), you disconfirm what you already know and notice what is new out there: "Wow, this looks so different today!" When you operate from Listening 3 (empathic listening), your perspective is redirected to seeing the situation through the eyes of another: "Wow, yes, now I really understand how you feel about it. I can sense it now, too." And finally, when you operate from Listening 4 (generative listening), you have gone through a subtle but profound change that has connected you to a deeper source of knowing, including the knowledge of your best future possibility and self (Otto Scharmer, Presencing Institute, in conversation).

Quite specifically, these are the practices that align with the four levels of listening and the Theory U awareness-based change model. This is the essence of how we move from "*me*" to "*we*" or ego- to eco-consciousness. The stages or levels of the listening practices follow the Theory U model. We first start with suspending any beliefs and sensing in to both our personal body and the earth body, and then extending the awareness in a close sensing practice to the relational field of resonance which might be called the social field or emerging social body.

It's in these co-creative awareness-based processes that we train our minds, hearts and wills to remain open, present and connected to all that is moving. Energy and information is flowing in and around us constantly; there are so many ways to identify experience and embrace conscious change-making practices and processes, rather than stay stuck. "Corona time" and the mystery of our shared emerging future are helping us embrace our shared humanity as we learn to let go of our own ego orientation or beliefs about what is supposed to happen next. Learning to rest in the moment is where the energy of connection, safety and meaning emerges, from our shared field of consciousness, collective awareness and emerging collective will.

The images shared here demonstrate that process and are deeply imprinted in my creative way of eliciting the deepest aspects, perhaps the soul and spirit aspects of each of these individuals as they landed in an embodied presence and then evoked a particular journey that illustrates, illuminates rather, their particular Yoga Radical journey of moving from "*me*" to "*we*."

The stories reveal a current or a reality that emerged in our conversation space; they were not prepared in advance—it's all a primary and spontaneous co-creative pre-reflective space.

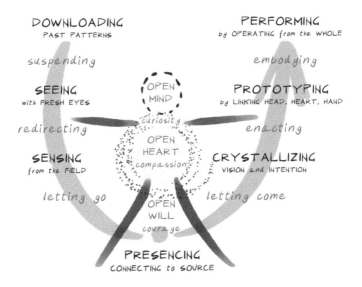

Theory U: Seven Ways of Attending and Co-shaping
The Essentials of Theory U—www.ottoscharmer.com

DOWNLOADING
PAST PATTERNS

OBSERVE,
OBSERVE,
OBSERVE

ACT in an INSTANT
PROTOTYPE

RETREAT and REFLECT
ALLOW the INNER KNOWING to EMERGE

The U Process—Three Movements

The Essentials of Theory U—www.ottoscharmer.com

Remember, since this was initiated from a sense of expanding the yoga practice into the social field for the sake of increased wellbeing, specifically community healing and social activism, my particular interest is in seeing, feeling and sensing how each of these individuals describes their personal practice backgrounds, what they learned that helps them stay on path, on their sacred dharma path as they scaled up or lifted their awareness from a *"me"* place to a *"we"* place.

That journey is what each of the interviews reveals: the rich inner tapestry of the essence of each of these practitioners.

The basic structure of the interview follows the Theory U process: Co-initiation through conscious dialogue to establish the processes of Co-sensing, Co-presencing, Co-realizing or Co-crystallizing.

The five movements of the interview process are inspired by the Theory U awareness-based change model:

1. Initiation: suspending and seeing with fresh eyes.

2. Connecting: sensing from the field and letting go, making space for and attracting deeper states of awareness and being, connecting to Source.

3. Presencing and connecting to Source, landing and locating, asking "Who am I really, what is my work?," establishment of a grounded being-ness.

4. Letting come, making space for the emerging future as the crystallizing force of the vision and intention begins to come into form.

5. A new shape of an idea or project or potential system emerges, engaging the enacting, the prototyping and the energies of an actual co-creation coming alive as a co-evolutionary event.

This is a process of consciously unearthing something essential in order to rebirth, transform or transmute something that benefits the whole. This process is grounded in deeper contemplative practices that relate to performing results with others from the many sources of wisdom and deep non-dual awareness through time and space, individually and collectively. My intention is that this process and attendant embodied practices are felt in each of the curated narratives, as singular demonstrations of embodied presence practices, as each Yoga Radical broadcasts their sets of potential, each in their own unique manner to help dream our new world into being.

Background Bibliography

There are a great many ancient texts that sing the myriad songs of yoga, meditation and conscious leadership. However, they do not paint a complete picture.

In addition to ancient texts like the *Bhagavad Gita and Upanishads*, the *Hatha Yoga Pradipika* and the many translations of *The Yoga Sutras of Patanjali*, as well as the many variations of the teachings of Siddhartha Gautama, also known as the Buddha, there is a whole host of latter-day texts that have informed my journey. I have included them below and encourage you to seek some of them out. Further, in addition to guidance from sacred texts and necessary study with masters, remember to listen to the earth and stars and the many myriad forces moving through and around you. This is our time to welcome the portals of potency, our continuing pathway of connection to the sacred.

Angelou, M. (1979) *I Know Why the Caged Bird Sings*. New York, NY: Random House.

Baldwin, J. (1984) *Notes of a Native Son*. Boston, MA: Beacon Press.

Bateson, G. (1972) *Steps to an Ecology of Mind*. Chicago & London: The University of Chicago Press.

Bird, K. (2018) *On Scribing: A Social Art of the Twentieth Century*. Massachusetts: PI Press.

Bohm, D. (2003) *The Essential David Bohm* (L. Nichol, Ed.). London, England: Routledge.

Bohm, D. (2012) *On Creativity* (2nd ed.). London, England: Routledge.

Bohm, D. (2014) *On Dialogue*. London, England: Routledge.

Brook, P. (2008) *The Empty Space*. London, England: Penguin. (First published 1968.)

Buhner, S. H. (2014) *Plant Intelligence and the Imaginal Realm: Beyond the Doors of Perception into the Dreaming of Earth*. Rochester, NY: Bear & Company.

Burbea, R. (2015) *The Seeing that Frees: Meditations on Emptiness and Dependent Arising*. Hermès Amara Publications.

Campbell, J. (1988) *Hero with a Thousand Faces*. London, England: Abacus.

David-Neel, A. (1983) *My Journey to Lhasa*. London, England: Virago Press.

Denning, P. J. and Dunham, R. (2012) *The Innovator's Way: Essential Practices for Successful Innovation*. Cambridge, MA: MIT Press.

Flowers, B. S., Scharmer, C. O., Jaworski, J. and Senge, P. M. (2011) *Presence: Exploring Profound Change in People, Organizations and Society*. London, England: Nicholas Brealey Publishing.

George, J. (1995) *Asking for the Earth: Waking up to the Spiritual/Ecological Crisis*. London, England: Element Books.

Gladwell, M. (2006) *Blink: The Power of Thinking Without Thinking*. Harlow, England: Penguin Books.

Gurdjieff, G. I. (1985) *Meetings with Remarkable Men*. London, England: Penguin Classics.

Gurdjieff, G. I. (1991) *Life is Real Only Then, When "I Am."* New York, NY: Penguin Group.

Hayashi, A. (2020) *Social Presencing Theatre: The Art of the True Move*. Massachusetts: PI Press.

Jaworski, J. (2012) *Source: The Inner Path of Knowledge Creation*. San Francisco, CA: Berrett-Koehler Publishers.

Jung, C. G. (1995) *Memories, Dreams, Reflections* (R. Winston & C. Winston, Trans.). London, England: Fontana Press.

Kabat-Zinn, J. (2004) *Wherever You Go, There You Are: Mindfulness Meditation for Everyday Life*. London, England: Piatkus Books.

Kimmerer, R. W. (2015) *Braiding Sweetgrass: Indigenous Wisdom, Scientific Knowledge and the Teachings of Plants*. Minneapolis, MN: Milkweed Editions.

Kingsley, P. (2004) *Reality*. Point Reyes Station, CA/Salisbury, England/Bern, Switzerland: Golden Sufi Center.

Maturana Rumesin, H. and Varela, F. J. (1992) *The Tree of Knowledge*. Boston, MA: Shambhala Publications.

Middleton, A. (2020) *A Wayfinder's Wanderings*. Lulu.

Ouspensky, P. D. (1988) *In Search of the Miraculous: Fragments of an Unknown Teaching*. Pyrmont, Australia: Law Book Co. of Australasia.

Petitmengin, C. (2006) "Describing one's subjective experience in the second person: An interview method for the science of consciousness." *Phenomenology and the Cognitive Sciences 5*, 229–269.

Presencing.org (n.d.). Retrieved January 25, 2021, from Presencing.org website: www.presencing.org/aboutus.

Roche, L. (2014) *The Radiant Sutras: 112 Gateways to the Yoga of Wonderland Delight*. Louisville, CO: Sounds True.

Salzmann, J. de (2011) *The Reality of Being*. Boston, MA: Shambhala Publications.

Scharmer, C. O. (2008) *Theory U: Leading from the Future as it Emerges* (1st ed.). Leipzig, Germany: Meine Verlag.

Scharmer, C. O. & Kaufer, K. (2013) *Leading from the Emerging Future*. San Francisco, CA: Berrett-Koehler.

Senge, P. M. (2006) *The Fifth Discipline: The Art and Practice of the Learning Organization*. New York, NY: Image Books.

Senge, P., Kruschwitz, N., Laur, J. and Smith, B. (2010) *The Necessary Revolution: How Individuals and Organizations Are Working Together to Create a Sustainable World*. London, England: Nicholas Brealey Publishing.

Sheldrake, M. (2020) *Entangled Life: How Fungi Make Our Worlds, Change Our Minds and Shape Our Futures*. London, England: Penguin Random House.

Siegel, D. J. (2008) *Neurobiology of "We."* Louisville, CO: Sounds True.

Siegel, D. J. (2010) *Mindsight: The New Science of Personal Transformation*. New York, NY: Bantam Books.

Steiner, R. (2004) *Start Now: Meditation Instructions, Meditations, Prayers, Verses for the Dead, Karma and Other Spiritual Practices for Beginners and Advanced Students*. Great Barrington, MA: SteinerBooks.

Torbert, W. R. and Cook-Greuter, S. R. (2004) *Action Inquiry: The Secret of Timely and Transforming Leadership*. San Francisco, CA: Berrett-Koehler.

Chögyam Trungpa (2008) *True Perception: The Path of Dharma Art*. (Judith L. Lief, Ed.). Boston, MA: Shambhala Publications.

Yeomans, T. (2020) *Holy Fire: The Process of Soul Awakening*. Shelbourne Falls, MA: Booksmyth Press.

Thresholds of Blue Timelessness

(what was said as we checked out, an archetypal poem)

I

Even if I am just an "emergent"
attempting to articulate,
to speak the words,

being in your space and
seeing something
is amazing.

Staying present
to
knowing
we don't have to teach.

It's in the allowing.

II

Now
I know why
you were listening to me.

We've got some threads
from staying present
to our common threads,

opening circles
of connection
on the grid.